TEENS WHO HURT

TEENS WHO HURT

*Clinical Interventions to Break
the Cycle of Adolescent Violence*

● ● ●

KENNETH V. HARDY
TRACEY A. LASZLOFFY

THE GUILFORD PRESS
New York London

© 2005 The Guilford Press
A Division of Guilford Publications, Inc.
72 Spring Street, New York, NY 10012
www.guilford.com

Printed in the United States of America

This book is printed on acid-free paper.

Last digit is print number: 9 8 7 6 5 4 3 2 1

Library of Congress Cataloging-in-Publication Data
Hardy, Kenneth V.
  Teens who hurt: clinical interventions to break the cycle of
adolescent violence / Kenneth V. Hardy, Tracey A. Laszloffy.
     p. cm.
  ISBN 1-57230-749-8 (cloth)
  Includes bibliographical references (p.) and index.
  1. Violence in adolescence—Prevention.   2. Juvenile delinquency—
Prevention.   3. Adolescent psychotherapy.   I. Laszloffy, Tracey A.
II. Title
  RJ506.V56 H37 2005
  618.92′ 8582 22

                                            2004026675

About the Authors

Kenneth V. Hardy, PhD, is a professor of family therapy at Syracuse University and is Director of the Eikenberg Institute for Relationships in New York. He is the former Director of the Center for Children, Families, and Trauma at the Ackerman Institute for the Family in New York. Dr. Hardy has provided training and consultation for working with troubled children and youth throughout the United States, Europe, and Asia. His work has been featured on *The Oprah Winfrey Show, 20/20, Dateline NBC*, PBS, and the Discovery Health Channel. Dr. Hardy maintains a private practice in New York.

Traccy A. Laszloffy, PhD, is a relationship therapist who specializes in working with troubled adolescents and their families. Currently she maintains a private practice in Connecticut, and prior to this, she directed the Marriage and Family Therapy master's program at Seton Hill University in Greensburg, Pennsylvania. Dr. Laszloffy has published extensively, and she routinely provides training and consultation to organizations that work with at-risk youth.

Acknowledgments

We want to thank several people for the contributions they made to this book. Foremost among them are the adolescents and their families who so courageously opened their hearts to us, trusted us with their stories, and allowed us to share parts of their lives with others. We remain grateful to them for their faith in us and for the risks that each of them took in allowing us into their world. They taught us a great deal, and without their courage and their confidence in us we never would have been able to develop the model we present in this book—hence, this book would never have been possible.

In addition to the adolescents themselves and their families, we want to acknowledge the countless educators, social service professionals, and other concerned adults who have devoted themselves to nurturing and supporting young people. Many of them have struggled alone for years with minimal institutional support while extending themselves to kids who so desperately need their help. Often at great personal and professional costs, these individuals have challenged the systems they work in to see the good in kids who do bad things and to create opportunities for healing and growth. They too have taught us so much about the challenges facing adolescents who turn to violence and how we can best help these kids.

Thank you to our colleagues who have been there for us on countless occasions to discuss difficult cases and to listen and offer feedback to our ideas while we were in the process of developing and refining them. And, of course, thank you to our families for their patience with us when we have felt tired, disheartened, and in despair, and for the ways in which they stood by us as we labored to commit to paper the work that has been the focus of so much of our time, energy, and attention.

Contents

Introduction

About 10 years ago we began doing therapy with troubled and often violent adolescents. As our work developed we began to receive invitations to consult with schools and communities throughout the United States who were struggling with aggression, bullying, and violence among young people. Guided by the premise that all people have the potential to be violent, the question that most nagged at us was: Why do some resort to violence while others do not? We wanted to understand what factors underpin this problem, and we wanted to develop strategies for counteracting those influences. From the many hours we spent talking with countless teenagers and their families in therapy and with the adolescent victims and perpetrators of violence in schools and communities across the United States, gradually our model for understanding and addressing adolescent violence emerged.

Our model assumes that indeed we all have the potential to be violent, but what seems to differentiate those who actualize this potential from those who do not is the interaction of four aggravated factors: devaluation, erosion of community, dehumanized loss, and rage. In this book we discuss each of these factors, explain what they mean, and outline strategies for how parents, teachers, therapists, and other concerned adults can take specific actions to address and ultimately reduce this violence.

Fifteen years ago, this book probably would not have attracted the attention of most of America. While urban, poor communities of color were well versed in the prevalence, consequences, and need to attend to adolescent violence, prior to the mid-1990s most of America had not yet recognized the seriousness of this problem. When we first began working with violent teens almost 10 years ago, adolescent violence was just beginning to capture the attention of the nation, and at that time a book like this probably would have garnered much interest. Presently, in the aftermath of 9/11 and with the country's anxious focus on war and terrorism, the problem of adolescent violence may seem less important or even passé to many Americans.

Much like a child with attention-deficit/hyperactivity disorder (ADHD), as a society our attention shifts rapidly from one arousing and captivating set of stimuli to another. We have a hard time focusing for very long on any particular issue. In our rapidly paced, technologically advanced, super-speed society, we are all bombarded with a relentless stream of viscerally arousing, quickly moving stimuli. We live in an age when *CNN Headline News* has us "around the world in 60 minutes," and in those 60 minutes multiple focal points are broadcast simultaneously, all beckoning for our attention. From the main news features, to the headline news streaking across the bottom of the screen, to the sports report appearing in one corner and the weather report appearing in another, we are subjected to a perpetual blast of competing demands for our focus. With so much competition for our attention, each byte of information must be presented in increasingly provocative, sexy, colorful, tantalizing, and shocking ways if it is to have any chance of capturing our gaze. And even when a stimulus has caught our attention, in the final analysis, no one is capable of holding on to it for very long.

Adolescent violence has been a serious problem in this country for decades, but it wasn't until the late 1990s—when the face of the violence shifted from urban streets to suburban and rural schools, from black and Latino kids to white kids, from those who were poor to those who were middle-class or affluent, and even from boys to girls—that this problem attracted national attention. For a period of time, these shootings and the broader, deeper problem they pointed to were shocking to most Americans. But the public's attention cannot remain focused for very long on any particular issue.

In late 2001 the media found a new crisis to rally around. In the wake of the 9/11 tragedy, and in this new era of war and terrorism, our attention has been diverted from the problem of adolescent violence. But this shift in focus should not be confused with amelioration of the problem. To the contrary, far too many young people across the United States continue to suffer from the trauma that both leads to and that flows from violence. Adolescent violence is now, as it was 5 years ago, and 5 years before that, a serious problem that threatens the health and welfare of our young people.

Currently we are living in a period when the anxiety created by the perception of a terrorist threat and the growing list of Americans killed in Iraq make it hard for many of us focus on the problems of bullying, the threat of school shootings, and other forms of youth violence. Many of us are armed with a heightened sense of alertness and guardedness that is directed at noticing and being prepared to defend against an external terrorist threat. For most Americans, the perception is that the greatest threat exists somewhere "out there" rather than right here in our midst.

While the issue of adolescent violence may no longer arouse the same interest or fervor that it did before 9/11, Al Q'aeda, Iraq, and the war on terrorism, for those families and communities that have been assaulted directly by this violence, the retreat from a broad national consciousness about and commitment to addressing this problem is often painful. As one mother wrote to us following a workshop we presented on youth violence:

"I attended your workshop as a mother who lost her 15-year-old son at the hands of another 15-year-old boy with a gun. What enrages me as much as the senseless violence that took my son's life is the indifference our society has to the violence that infects an entire generation of our young people. We spend billions of dollars waging war in another nation, billions of dollars trying to fight the terrorists who want to destroy us. But what about what's happening right here in our families, our schools, and our backyards? I don't know what the reason is for the rampant violence among our kids, but I want to understand and I want to know that as a society we all notice and care about this problem as much as we care about addressing other horrors in the world. If we don't, then by the time we wipe out terrorism (if we do), there won't be much left here anyway."

As this mother's words reveal, the families and communities that are directly assaulted by adolescent violence realize the seriousness of this problem as 7intensely as our nation feels the threat of terrorism and the danger of war. But collectively our focus has shifted, and this problem no longer attracts the type of recognition that it needs to garner if we truly are to address and overcome it. It may well be that this issue will not recapture public interest until there is another Columbine massacre, or worse. Certainly, we hope it does not have to come to that, and this is what we hope to accomplish with this book. It is our intention to help readers understand the scope, nature, and dangers of the phenomenon of adolescent violence. But more importantly, we hope to provide a framework to clarify why this violence exists and offer specific strategies for what each of us can do individually and collectively to address and ultimately prevent it.

The current level of anxiety about terrorist violence and the increasing losses associated with the war in Iraq only intensify the likelihood and seriousness of youth violence. Young people today are living in an environment that is strained by the fear of trauma. Like the drive-by shooter who suddenly lurches around the corner in an unexpected moment, unloading a spray of bullets that randomly assaults anyone in the vicinity, terrorist attacks create a comparable fear rooted in the element of surprise and generalized victimization. American children today live in a society where they are held hostage by the threat of an impending attack. Those who live in this chronic state of tension, uncertainty, and aggression are more vulnerable to violence, because at some point it begins to feel commonplace and inevitable. When kids of any age can view beheadings of hostages over and over on the Internet, at some point they become numb to the horror and ugliness of this brutality. Violence—or the threat of it—becomes the norm rather than the exception, and this makes young people more likely to resort to it and more conditioned to tolerate it.

Living in a chronic state of threat fosters a hardness, a callousness toward pain—both one's own and that of others. It's a defense against pervasive stress, but if it persists long enough, with the deadening of feelings comes a loss of inhibition and even of fear itself. At some point a boldness emerges whereby a person can conceive of doing just about anything because there is a sense of having very little left to lose. This is the reality that poor children of color in urban war zones have lived with for decades. It's what so many Iraqi, Chechen, Sudanese, and Palestinian children endure. After living in a state of constant threat, of constantly anticipating or actually being the target of another's aggression, when so much has been lost, at some point people become conditioned to the horror of violence, which breeds aggression. It's built into human biology that in response to a threat we either "fight or flee." For those who don't believe there is anyplace to flee to and for those who regard fleeing as a sign of weakness, or for those who have lost so much that there is a sense of having very little left to lose, an aggressive instinct is honed. In this way, living with the ever-present threat of harm nurtures a level of aggressiveness in young people that can only increase the risk of youth violence.

Another potential consequence of living in these times is that such circumstances tend to exacerbate ethnic and religious divisions. The nascent trend in bullying is no longer so much about "the bad kids" picking on the "the good kids," or the "tough guy" who muscles "the weakling." Instead, it more reflective of "blue-blood kids" targeting kids who are believed to be Muslims or immigrants. There is so much intense hatred and suspicion that has been generated toward anyone who appears "Middle Eastern" or Islamic or simply "foreign" that this creates a climate that breeds bigotry, ignorance, and aggression. More and more we are hearing about kids who, because they don't seem "American enough" or "Christian enough," have been targeted by other kids who see them as "outsiders" and therefore as potentially unsafe and suspicious. Certainly Muslim children routinely are subjected to bullying from other kids who see them as "terrorists." But also children who simply look Middle Eastern in some way, irrespective of what their actual ethnic or religious identity is, are often targets of bullying. We have heard accounts of attacks upon Jewish kids wearing yarmulkes and Mexican American children who were mistakenly assumed to be "Arabs." In these instances the attackers are responding to a conditioned hatred against anyone who appears to be "other."

What is important to understand is that the trend in bullying, with its strong xenophobic undercurrent, is reflective of what young people today are learning from the adults around them. Kids mimic the adults in their lives, adults whom they hear making bigoted and hateful comments about those whom they perceive as "others." The promotion of "other" from the broader political sphere makes it possible for us to distance from the suffering that violence creates, which increases the likelihood of more violence. When any living being becomes "other" in our eyes, it becomes easier to inflict violence upon that individual with little hesitation or remorse. We are conditioned to not relate to the "other" as someone like ourselves, with feelings, interests, or connections to family. Our compassion is short-circuited, and at that point violence is not only possible but highly likely. This is what happened in Abu Ghraib where U.S. military prison guards piled up the naked bodies of Iraqi prisoners to beat and humiliate them for amusement. The acts were possible because in the eyes of the guards the Iraqi prisoners were "other."

Another consequence of the times we currently live in is that our strained circumstances send a powerful message to young people sanctioning violence as a solution to problems. Children learn from what they observe. Hence, we may preach to them about the value of nonviolence and peace, but if they see us behaving in ways that legitimize the use of force as a way of "getting what we want," this is what they will learn. In this time of war, our young people are especially vulnerable to learning that aggression is a solution. While they may hear spirited debates among adults ranging from their parents to political candidates, at the end of the day they live in a society actively engaged in the use of militarism as a method of managing a difficult situation. They also hear the often cited rationale for this force which is that "we have to get them before they get us." Such a message increases the likelihood that young people will resort to violence as a way of managing their problems and as a defense against their fear of being hurt. Hence, now, during these times of terrorism and war, when the fear of violence looms so ominously across this nation in a broader, more generalized way, now more than ever each of us must be attuned to, concerned about, and committed to addressing both potential and actual violence among adolescents.

Of course, we don't want to suggest that all is bleak. While terrorism and war having numbing and damaging effects, for sure, there also is a bright side that should be acknowledged. During times of great stress and turmoil people get motivated to take action. We live in a society that tends to be reactive rather than proactive. As a result, we are most likely to act with intention when confronted with a crisis. Our current state is just the type of crisis that can inspire organized peace-based activities. Feeling the threat of what might happen if we don't find less aggressive methods for managing the dilemmas we face, families and communities around the country are finding creative ways to develop nonviolent alternatives. We have talked with families that have responded to the increased violence in the world by initiating family conversations about how people can find diplomatic solutions to divisive conflicts. We have had the privilege of learning about schools and communities that have spearheaded initiatives designed to advance constructive approaches for responding to both global and local conflicts. And among adolescents, as often as we hear stories of violence, trauma, and pain, we also have heard stories of hope and healing, of young people who have pushed back against the pressure of fear and aggression through loving, peace-based collaborations. In

examples like these we see the seeds of hope that are directly reflective of an underlying thrust of this book, namely, that it is incumbent
on each of us as adults to find ways to see the good in the bad, to
replace cynicism with optimism, replace fear with courage, bitterness
with forgiveness, and to challenge despair with hopeful possibilities.
Throughout this volume we argue that young people will learn from
what they see us do, and, as we live in times of extreme tension and
aggression, now more than ever we must provide young people with
living examples of how to promote healing and practice hopeful, positive action to counteract the pressure to succumb to violence.

PART I
. . . . . .
The Model

CHAPTER 1

● ● ● ● ● ● ●

Adolescent Violence in a Sociocultural Context

We were captivated immediately by the bright, cherubic face and the sweet, gap-toothed smile. His smooth, pinkish complexion, unblemished by acne, and his deep dark brown eyes sparkled with the glow of innocence and the promise of the best that life had yet to offer. The image of an adorable, then 5-year-old Andrew Golden contrasted starkly with the camouflage military fatigues he was wearing and the rifle that was balanced somewhat awkwardly against his small shoulder. The odd juxtapositions reflected in this photo make it easy to see why the editors of *Newsweek* included it as part of an April 1998 cover story on the proliferation of school shootings across the United States.

The *Newsweek* article that featured Andrew had nothing to do with any of our idealized, heart-warming notions of childhood. There was no mention of high academic achievement, outstanding accomplishments in sports, noble deeds or acts of community service. Instead, Andrew's place, in *Newsweek* and in history, has been defined by an act that for many of us is incomprehensible: the premeditated and vicious mass slaying of his classmates at Westside Middle School in Jonesboro, Arkansas.

The significance of Andrew's story lies not in its uniqueness but rather in its growing banality. The wave of school shootings perpetrated by adolescents is but one example of the ways in which we, as a nation, have been assaulted by a growing epidemic of adolescent violence. While violence of any kind, irrespective of the perpetrator's age, is disturbing, the notion of youthful aggressors strikes a particularly

11

sensitive chord within many adults. Our commonly held beliefs regarding the innocence and purity of childhood make it especially hard to comprehend the extreme acts of brutality that a growing number of young people are committing.

According to noted Cornell University professor James Garbarino (1999), the current epidemic of youth violence has followed an evolutionary course that parallels most epidemics. These begin "among the most vulnerable segments of the population and then work their way outward, like ripples in a pond. These vulnerable populations don't cause the epidemic. Rather, *their disadvantaged position makes them a good host for the infection*" (pp. 15–16, emphasis in original). This pattern is evident with regard to youth violence in America. "The first wave of lethal youth violence in schools peaked in the 1992–1993 school year, when fifty people died, mostly in urban schools and involving low-income minority youth. . . . We are now in Stage Two, the spread of youth violence throughout American society" (p. 16).

It is interesting to note that, until recently, most Americans didn't seem to notice or express concern about the problem of youth violence. Ten years ago, youth violence did not garner national headlines or arouse legislators and social scientists urgently to seek out answers and solutions. Anyone who lived in a major city like Washington, DC, Philadelphia, Detroit, Chicago, Miami, Los Angeles, or New York was probably attuned to the issue of youth violence as a local phenomenon, but the subject received little attention from the national media. The slaughter of 50 people in schools during 1992–1993 did *not* result in a White House Conference on Youth Violence. The reason in part, as suggested by Garbarino, is linked to the fact that initially most of the killings were consistent with stage 1. In other words, they occurred among the most vulnerable communities in America: inner-city communities where the perpetrators and the victims were largely low-income African American and Latino youth. As long as the problem of youth violence was concentrated within poor communities of color, racism and classism mitigated against mainstream America's noticing or attending to this violence in any meaningful way. But this changed significantly in 1998.

In 1998 there was a wave of school shootings committed by white middle-class boys in mostly white suburban communities. That was the start of the stage 2 period Garbarino described. It was also at that point that the issue of youth violence catapulted into the media spotlight and to the top of our political agenda. Today most of America is obsessed with understanding the parameters of the problem: What contributes to violence among teens and, most significantly, what is the antidote to this epidemic? These are the questions that we will grapple with in this volume. Not only will we consider the nature and magnitude of the problem, but also we will engage you in an in-depth examination of the factors that underpin adolescent violence. We will share with you four factors that we believe are critical in leading to youth violence. Most importantly, we will make specific recommendations for how each of us can work to intervene in the lives of angry adolescents, and ultimately to prevent this violence.

WHAT WE MEAN BY "VIOLENCE"

Violence involves a willful action (or inaction) that results in the intentional infliction of harm or injury. Using this definition, traditional examples of violence involve physical acts of aggression that one person directs against another. Yet, our definition is deliberately broad to allow for various "nontraditional" circumstances that we believe also constitute violence. There are three such circumstances that we wish to focus on. First, we believe that violence includes intentionally harmful actions that a person directs against him- or herself. Hence, we consider suicide to be as much an act of violence as homicide. In addition to this, Alderman (1997) coined the term "self-inflicted violence" (SIV) to describe situations in which persons set out to cause harm and injury to themselves without any obvious suicidal intent. For example, persons who burn, cut, or otherwise mutilate themselves are engaging in SIV.

Second, we believe that violence is not limited to the interpersonal level and that it is also inflicted at the broader social level as well. Therefore, we believe that war, genocide, slavery, and all manifestations of sociocultural oppression—whether it's racism, sexism, homophobia, or poverty—are acts of violence. Each of these acts invariably involves some form of domination coupled with inequities based on differential access to power, influence, and resources. When these conditions coexist in human relationships, regardless of the level, violence is inevitable.

Finally, we believe that violence can be perpetrated passively through acts of omission. In other words, if a person is aware of a violent act and refuses to take specific action to intervene and prevent this occurrence, we believe this person is "an accomplice." For example, a mother who is aware that her husband is sexually abusing their daughter and does nothing to intervene ultimately shares the blame for the husband's continuing violence. We realize this last point may stretch the average reader's comfort zone, but we want to make this point now because it underpins the spirit of activism that is reflected in this book.

PREVALENCE OF ADOLESCENT VIOLENCE

Are the Andrew Goldens merely a fluke phenomenon or, rather, evidence of a significant and alarming change in the wider culture of adolescence? According to FBI statistics, youth under the age of 21 account for nearly one-third of the overall homicide rate (Snyder, 2000). Comparatively speaking, the rate of homicides committed by U.S. youth is eight times higher than it is in other industrialized nations (Centers for Disease Control and Prevention, 1997). Moreover, juveniles under age 18 were involved in 27% of all serious violent victimizations, including 14% of sexual assaults, 30% of robberies, and 27% of aggravated assaults (Snyder & Sickmund, 1999). According to the Office of Juvenile Justice Delinquency and Prevention (1997), 28% of teens carry weapons, and during the last 10 years, weapons-related offenses among youth between the ages of 10 and 17 have doubled. Also, within the past decade, the rate of aggravated assaults committed by adolescents has increased by 64%.

In recent years the number of youth involved in gangs has increased dramatically, and where there are gangs there is violence. The reality is that gangs contribute greatly to the escalation in homicides, aggravated assaults, rapes, and other forms of violence that adolescents commit (Hampton, Jenkins, & Gullotta, 1996; Thornberry, & Burch, 1997). Ironically, many adolescents join gangs as a form of protection *against* violence. As one adolescent male told us when asked why he was part of a gang, "The gang is a cover. Without this cover I would have been dead a long time ago. So, whatever I have to do to keep this cover, I'll do it. It's as simple as get or be gotten." This boy's chilling words reflect the reality that gangs and violence are inextricably intertwined. Many young people may join gangs because they provide a buffer against violence, but in exchange for this buffer members are often required to commit crimes that lead to further violence. It is an unending vicious cycle.

In terms of violence directed inwardly, the data are equally distressing. During the past 30 years the adolescent suicide rate has increased 300%. During the last decade the suicide rate for children between the ages of 10 and 14 has tripled. Among college-age youth, suicide is the third leading cause of death. Girls attempt suicide four to eight times more often than boys, although boys succeed four times more often because they tend to use more lethal means (e.g., firearms, auto crashes, hanging) (Centers for Disease Control and Prevention, 1998). With regard to race, the statistics are equally alarming. According to a Centers for Disease Control and Prevention study, there has been a 114% increase in suicides among black males aged 10–19 from 1980 through 1995, a larger figure than among any other group. For black males in the 10–14 age group, the rate of increase was 233%, compared with a 146% increase for white males in the same age category. Although we have no scientific data to support such a claim, it has always been our belief, based on our work, that many of the young children of color caught up in the crossfire of urban violence have been those with the most pronounced suicidal ideations.

SIV is the intentional act of physically hurting one's self. Behaviors can range from hitting or bruising oneself, to cutting, burning, interfering with the healing of wounds, excessive nail biting or hair pulling, and the breaking of bones. Perhaps because the idea of purposefully hurting and mutilating one's own body is so hard to imagine, SIV has not received the public attention it warrants. Given that most acts of SIV begin in late adolescence and peak in the early 20s, we believe any study of adolescent violence must take this phenomenon into consideration. "It has been estimated that approximately 960,000 to 1.8 million individuals in the United States engage in these behaviors" (Alderman, 1997, p. 188), and most of them are older adolescents and very young adults.

Priya, a 16-year-old girl, ritualistically burned her arms and legs with a cigarette every few months. She never allowed anyone to see her uncovered skin, which she kept hidden beneath long black skirts and long-sleeved black sweaters or shirts. Sheila was 14 when she began regularly cutting herself with a razor blade. When her wounds began to heal she often rewounded herself by picking at the scabs until they bled. Mark, a 17-year-old male, admitted to throwing himself down a flight of stairs in the hope of breaking an arm or leg. When this failed, he resorted to breaking his finger with a hammer. These are all examples of SIV.

In addition to self-mutilation, substance abuse and eating disorders are other ways in which adolescents often make themselves the targets of their own self-directed violence. Despite widespread drug education programs in the media and in schools, far too many adolescents develop abusive relationships with substances, regularly placing their health and safety in jeopardy. In terms of eating disorders, anorexia nervosa, which involves self-starvation, is most common among females between the ages of 13 and 20. Bulimia nervosa refers to cyclical patterns of bingeing and purging (e.g., self-induced vomiting, laxative or diuretic abuse, excessive exercise) and it is most common among older female adolescents and young women in their early 20's (Gordon, 1990). It has been estimated that after puberty 5–10 million girls and women are afflicted with anorexia and bulimia nervosa (Shisslak, Crago, & Estes, 1995).

YOUTH AS VICTIMS: THE CYCLE OF VIOLENCE

Why are so many youth turning to violence against others or themselves? Many therapists point to the statistics that show that many youth perpetrators of violence are also victims of it. Approximately 13% of children are victims of neglect, while 11% are victims of abuse (U.S. Department of Health and Human Services, 2003). While this is certainly not the sole reason for teen violence, there is obviously a cyclical relationship that can and often does exist between those who are victims of violence and those who are perpetrators. While not all abused and neglected children become aggressive and violent themselves, there is a strong positive correlation between being the victim of child maltreatment and developing aggressive and violent patterns of behavior. As evidenced in a longitudinal study conducted by Wisdom (1992), adolescents who had been abused or neglected as children were significantly more likely to be arrested for violence crimes as juveniles.

Children are exposed to violence not only within their homes but also in the outside world. Among children living in high-crime neighborhoods, more than one-third have witnessed a homicide by the time they turned 15 (Bell, 1991; Garbarino, 1995). A study of first and second graders living in Washington, DC, revealed that 45% had witnessed a mugging, 31% had witnessed a shooting, and 39% had seen a dead body (Cooley-Quille, Turner, & Beidel, 1995). In Chicago, since 1974, there has been a 400% increase in the rate of serious assaults that occur in public places. The conditions in cities like DC and Chicago are mirrored throughout the United States. More than 70% of high school students report that they have witnessed a serious assault in some location other than in their homes. In fact, 36% of assaults and 40% of robberies reported by people between the ages of 12 and 19 occurred within schools.

The level of violence that exists within communities contributes to an atmosphere of fear and insecurity for young people. Children and adolescents learn that the world is not a safe place, and the sense of threat they feel makes them suspicious, untrusting, and prone to violence as a means of self-protection. Citing several studies Allen (1994) reported that a fear of being kidnapped is a number one concern among children. Global events such as terrorism and war have also left an increasing number of children feeling unsafe and uneasy about their future.

In many cases, the level of threat and lack of safety that young people experience is most severe within urban communities that are ravaged by a confluence of social ills and injustices that undermine an overall sense of harmony and stability. Within such environments, fear, aggression, and a lack of safety become self-reinforcing. The more people feel at risk, the more likely they are to engage in behaviors that further undermine their safety. We have spoken to hundreds of young people who consistently report that they join gangs or carry guns not because they revel in violence, but as a form of protection. They perceive their environment as dangerous and threatening. Moreover, they don't trust that adults can or will be able to keep them safe from harm. In response to their overwhelming sense of imminent harm, many are driven to extreme courses of action out of fear and desperation, and tragically these actions often exacerbate the existing climate of peril.

The lack of safety is not limited to the most vulnerable communities in our nation. Children living within neighborhoods and attending schools that were once thought to be immune from the epidemic of widespread violence are also increasingly unsafe. In suburban and small-town communities across the country, children hear about, personally observe, or are directly victimized by drive-by shootings, random street violence, and other forms of public violence. One 11-year-old-boy we spoke with who attended an elementary school that was considered a model school within his state told us he carried a knife to protect himself from three other boys who had been taunting him for months. Recently they had started telling him that one day when he least expected it they were going to jump him, drag him into the woods, tie him up, and leave him there to die.

As quoted by Garbarino (1995):

> It does not take much violence and terror to set a tone of threat. . . .
> Memory of the emotions of trauma does not decay; it remains fresh.
> Once you have the feeling of danger, it takes very little new threat to sustain it. Many children learn to fear violence in the world around them.
> Whether they literally become the targets of violence, their fear is realistic—to some degree this fear is grounded in reality. (p. 65)

Social violence is not simply people with guns shooting at one another. There is a subtle form of harm being done every moment to the psyches and physical well-being of youth who live in poverty. The 20% of our nation's children who live in households at or under the poverty level are victims of this social violence. Poor children who go to school suffering from the wrenching pangs of hunger or the throbbing pain of decaying teeth are victims of the violence of poverty. Sadly, our society turns a blind eye to the plight of poor children. While we are able to leverage tax cuts for the rich and grant generous corporate subsidies, poor children are denied access to basic health-care and adequate nutrition. In this sense, as a nation, we are guilty of perpetrating violence against economically disadvantaged children.

The occurrence and effects of social violence are difficult to assess. Often the violence of sociocultural oppression occurs at the institutional level, where it assaults entire groups of people in a broad-sweeping manner over a period of time. For example, children of color are victimized by institutional racism, while little girls of all races are assaulted by institutional sexism. Gay, lesbian, and bisexual youth are assaulted by institutionalized homophobia and heterosexism that lead to things like constant assumptions of heterosexuality, the failure of the media to portray gay life in a positive manner, and the social acceptability of gay-bashing in schools, on TV and on the playground. Exposure to the seemingly small and "benign" indignities of institutionalized "isms" on an almost daily basis involves a slow, persistent conditioning process that silently but methodically assaults the psyches and souls of children who share membership in socially devalued groups. At the very least, these expressions create a climate of intolerance and hatred that often sets the stage for more overt acts of interpersonal violence directed against those who hold membership in oppressed groups.

The vicious slaying of young Matthew Shepard was a painful example of homophobic violence on the interpersonal level. While the

Shepard murder captured media attention, similar incidents are all too common across the country. While we were conducting a workshop in Illinois, a participant shared with us an incident in which two white boys who were members of a white supremacist group attacked a young African American boy. Not only did they beat the boy, they also carved the word "nigger" into his chest with a knife. Consider also the 1999 shooting massacre at Columbine High School in Littleton, Colorado. Eric Harris and Dylan Klebold, both of whom were white, murdered 13 people, all of whom were white except for one, Isaiah Shoels, an African American boy. We raise the issue of race because of the role it played in the murder of Shoels, who was referred to as "a nigger" by the shooters as he was being murdered. While Harris and Klebold were intent on committing indiscriminate murder, they specifically targeted Shoels because he was black. The murder of Shoels was just like the other 12 murders committed by the two assassins in most respects, but it also was unique in that it was a racially motivated act of violence.

At the interpersonal level, sexism often leads to violence against girls in the form of sexual abuse. Sexism contributes to the notion that females of all ages are sexual objects who exist primarily to gratify male sexual desire and to affirm male dominance. Simply put, countless numbers of young people who hold membership in socially marginal groups are victimized by the violence of "the isms." Whether it's through institutionalized violence or violence that occurs on a more direct, interpersonal level, sociocultural oppression creates trauma and suffering in the lives of young people. Especially in light of the connection between exposure to violence and becoming violent, it is critical that we, as adults, take an active role in challenging and preventing all forms of violence in the lives of young people. But this is no easy task for any of us. While most of us are committed in principle to peace, in practice many of us engage in and support violence in countless ways that we rarely even recognize.

OUR CONFLICTING ATTITUDES TOWARD VIOLENCE

One thing that makes it difficult to deal with adolescent violence involves our society's conflicting attitudes about this issue. We, as a society, have an ambivalent relationship with violence. On the one hand, most of us claim to abhor it. Various popular slogans or sayings declare our moral aversion to violence, such as "violence only begets violence", "just turn the other cheek," or "love thy neighbor." But, on the other hand, we also seem to tolerate violence, as evidenced by the ways in which we often glorify it in the world around us. For example, our celebration of war memorials and the many film heroes who use guns, as well as the overwhelming percentage of Americans who favored bombing Afghanistan after the 9/11 tragedy, are all examples of our pro-violence disposition. As a society, we seem to live all too comfortably with our desires to achieve peace through violence, deter crime with violence, as well as punish and discipline our young with violence.

How can it be possible to simultaneously condemn and condone violence? Isn't that a contradiction? It is. Yet, this is a contradiction that most of us live with on a daily basis. One does not have to search very hard to find examples of how we, as individuals and as a society, are able to simultaneously condemn violence as a matter of principle but act in ways that support violence in practice. One such example of this can be found in the case of Andrew Golden.

At a very early age Andrew's father and grandfather had introduced him to guns. Not only did they make guns available to him, they also taught him how to use guns to stalk and ambush living beings. They referred to this activity as "hunting," which Jonesboro (AR) mayor Hubert Brodell described as an all-American family pastime: "[Hunting] is done by husband and wife, by father and son and daughter. This is a family activity."

Based on media reports, Andrew's family was horrified to learn after the fact that, in pursing his human quarry, Andrew crouched in the bushes, focused the viewfinder of his rifle upon his intended target, and shot several rounds of ammunition that killed and injured five of his classmates in the schoolyard. No one in his family condoned this behavior or suggested that they thought it was anything but a senseless act of violence. However, neither the town's mayor, Andrew's father, nor his grandfather considered it violence when Andrew stalked and shot a deer or a duck. From their perspective, when the targets are human, the action is violence, but when the target is a deer or a duck, it's something altogether different, namely, hunting.

The point here is not to debate the ethics of hunting animals but rather to draw attention to the potential contradiction between calling the hunting of animals a family pastime and the killing of humans the crime of murder. We are concerned that in the eyes of Andrew, at least, these clearly distinguishable activities became very blurred.

Andrew's grandmother vehemently argued that he was a gentle boy who "when he wasn't hunting animals, was trying to save and care for them." To his grandmother, this statement made sense. She offered as proof that Andrew loved animals the fact that when he wasn't killing them he was caring for them. But the key words are "when he's not killing them." How is this different from the abusive husband who, when he's not bashing his wife's face in, is kissing her? Do his acts of tenderness somehow erase his acts of brutality?

As individuals and as a society, we have an ambivalent attitude toward violence. Because of this ambivalence, young people are inundated with mixed messages about violence that simultaneously teach them to abhor it but also to glorify it. Moreover, as individuals and as a society, we protect ourselves from having to confront our contradictions by developing sophisticated rationalizations. When a particular act of violence is something we believe in and support, we find ways to justify it, to call it something other than violence. We have many of these sophisticated reconstructions: "war," "capital punishment," "corporal punishment" and "development." One of our favorites is "discipline."

We routinely see families in therapy where play among siblings results in one child suddenly reaching out and giving his or her brother or sister a swat across the arm or leg. Appearing slightly embarrassed and mildly irritated, a parent will often respond by saying "we don't tolerate hitting in this family" while simultaneously using the back of his or her hand to deliver the message to the arm or leg of the offending youngster.

While we believe that any form of hitting is an act of violence, we realize there are many who would not agree. Time and again we have had parents explain to us that it's different when they hit, versus when their children hit. They defend their hitting as a legitimate way of fulfilling their parental responsibility to discipline their children. As one mother said to us:

"There's a difference between abuse and disciplining. I'm using physical punishment to discipline my child and teach him how to act right. If I don't do it now, who knows what he'll end up doing when he's grown."

Certainly this parent, and the many others who believe the same thing, is entitled to her view. From our perspective, however, it is contradictory to use hitting as a way of enforcing a rule that forbids hitting. We believe that striking another living being *for any reason* is a form of violence. To call it something else (even "discipline") in situations where the hitter is an adult (even if solely trying to correct a child) is a sophisticated example of rationalization. Moreover, we see this as an indication of the ambivalent relationship so many of us have with violence.

In recent years our contradictory attitude toward violence has been exposed. Following the horrific terrorist attack on the United States on September 11, 2001, most Americans wanted to retaliate against our enemies. The air was thick with rhetoric calling for "striking back" and "kicking some ass." The rationale for the proposed aggression was that it constituted "justifiable defense." But isn't that what the terrorists probably told themselves as well? Did they not convince themselves that the United States was the great Satan—a corrupt, morally bankrupt, exploitative, and unjust bully of the world? Didn't they believe that their act of violence was justified because they viewed it as a form of retaliation against a vicious enemy? As self-anointed holy warriors, they probably rationalized civilian casualties as a necessary means to achieving their greater end. This is exactly the rationale used to justify bombing Afghanistan and the civilian casualties that resulted there. And it's the same rationale that was advanced to justify the war in Iraq and the thousands of Iraqi citizens who have been killed or maimed as a consequence.

How are we able to tolerate these contradictions? In part, it is important to understand that violence and aggression are basic to human nature. Despite the social norms and mores we have developed to deter violent behavior, deep within our physiology and psychology, violence is a part of all of us. We all have the potential to be violent. From an evolutionary perspective, aggressive behavior played a necessary role in the survival of our species. Since it is coded into our DNA, the aggressive impulse resides within each human being. Under the right set of circumstances, any one of us is capable of great violence.

Given the role that evolutionary biology plays in human aggression and violence, it isn't terribly surprising that so many of us find ways to express our aggressive impulses. Some of us hunt, join the military, or compete in sports with an aggressive orientation (e.g., boxing, ice hockey). Others of us experience this impulse vicariously. We become voyeurs in ritualistic displays of dominance and violence ranging from the WWE (World Wrestling Entertainment), to football, to rodeos, to movies and television shows that depict violence.

The value of these activities is that they allow us to gratify a natural impulse while simultaneously denying our relationship to violence. Because our social values are so strongly anti-violent, we have developed a diverse vocabulary we can use to call our aggression and violence something else. In this way, we don't have to confront the contradictions between our rhetoric and our realities. And in this way we are better able to live with the contradictions, because we don't see our positions as contradictory.

In instances when we are challenged to think critically about the social constructions we have devised to recast violence as "something else" that is more permissible and less toxic, we become angry. For example, we have had many heated debates with friends, family, and colleagues about whether or not football is violence. Those who deny its violence refer to it instead as a healthy competition based on shrewd strategy. And that it is . . . but it also involves violence. The violence is an essential part of what fills football stadiums. It this were not so, we could find ways to preserve the strategy and competition without the aggression. We could replace tackle football with touch football. But who could honestly imagine football fans around the country clamoring to see their favorite teams "touch" rather than "tackle." The idea seems absurd because on some level we understand that the thrill is not just in the strategy—it's in the slamming of bodies, the crunching of bones, and the pounding of flesh against flesh.

The danger inherent in our contradictory relationship with violence is that it's confusing for young people. They hear our rhetoric about the immorality of violence, but they also see how we, as adults, behave. Of course, most of us would deny that we personally condone violence or have any role in the creation or maintenance of our culture of violence. While many of us are inclined to indict television, movies, music, video games, and the Internet for encouraging violence, few of us are willing to acknowledge our individual role in creating and maintaining pro-violence messages. While few of us have the power to shape the extent to which violence is reflected in the media, we can choose to act in ways that challenge media-depicted violence. For example, we can have conversations with young people about the violence they inevitably observe through the media.

Most importantly, we can choose to live our personal lives in ways that challenge, rather than conspire with, the message that violence is acceptable. We can examine our beliefs and behaviors honestly and resist the urge to rationalize the ways in which even we support violence. We can recognize that, while our instinct for aggression may account for our survival in the past, our survival in the future hinges much more on our capacity to find nonaggressive and nonviolent means of coping with the challenges we face. With this understanding, we can resist our impulse to resort to aggression and violence and replace it with tactics of negotiation and diplomacy as a means of solving conflicts and acquiring necessary resources. In other words, we can begin by personally challenging ourselves to create greater congruence and harmony between what we believe in and what we actually do.

WHY SOME TURN VIOLENT AND SOME DON'T

Why do some children become violent and not others? Again and again in our work we have encountered this basic conundrum. Directly and indirectly, the lives of young people today are besieged by violence, and this increases the risk that they will in turn become violent toward themselves or others. Yet, not all do. In this volume we will examine the four aggravating factors we have found through our work that help us understand what makes some more likely than others to become violent themselves. And more importantly, we will share how our understanding of the four aggravating factors can be translated into practical strategies that can be used to stop violence and to prevent potential violence from actually occurring.

AGGRAVATING VERSUS ETIOLOGICAL FACTORS

Within the past decade, our work with violent teens has led to the development of a model that we use to conceptualize the anatomy of adolescent violence, and to inform our prevention and intervention strategies. This model helps us understand what leads to violence in the lives of teens. Moreover, because it also helps us to understand why some kids become violent and others do not, the most hopeful part of the model is that it gives us direction for how to address and ultimately prevent such violence.

We have found four aggravating factors to be closely tied to the phenomenon of adolescent violence. We use the term "aggravating", as opposed to "etiological," factors because we want to dispel the idea that these factors *cause* violence. Human behavior is complex. It is far too complex to establish neat and simple cause-and-effect relationships. Therefore, we use the term aggravating factors to emphasize that while the mix of these factors plays a critical role in adolescent violence, we are not suggesting that they cause violence.

The four aggravating factors are devaluation, disruption/erosion of community, the dehumanization of loss, and rage. It is the confluence of these four aggravating factors that we believe is located at the heart of what divides those who do from those who don't engage in violence. In reality, these four factors are connected inextricably. There is a synergy between them. Think of clothes in a dryer. When the dryer is in operation, it tosses the clothes inside around and around until eventually each of these seemingly separate pieces become fused in a dynamic swirl of color and texture. It is no longer possible to distinguish among the individual items because the tossing has merged all of the items beyond distinction. The four aggravating factors are interconnected in just this way. For example, devaluation often contributes to a disruption of community, and vice versa. Devaluation and the disruption of community are also forms of loss, and when losses remain unacknowledged this often contributes to a sense of devaluation. Whenever devaluation, disruption of community, and the dehumanization of loss co-occur, rage is an inevitable consequence. In a way, not all of the aggravating factors are on the same level because it is the presence of the first three that contributes to the last one (rage).

Rage is the "last step" before violence occurs. When rage develops within a person and there are few to no opportunities to express and channel rage constructively, the potential for violence increases exponentially. Of course, violence is not inevitable. The first three factors increase the risk of violence, but they do not always lead to violence. We have found that there are various ways to decrease the potential that the aggravating factors will lead to violence. Therefore, after describing each aggravating factor in detail in the first part of the book, in the second part we focus on describing specific strategies for addressing the factors and reducing the risk of violence.

OVERVIEW OF THE MODEL

Devaluation is the first aggravating factor in our model. Devaluation occurs when an individual or group's dignity and worth are assaulted or denigrated. Devaluation can arise in response to situational circumstances, such as abandonment, unemployment, or school failure. For example, consider the life circumstances of one our clients Delores.

Delores was put up for adoption when she was 3 days old because her birth mother, at age 17, was unprepared for motherhood. Her adoptive parents, who told her from the beginning she was adopted, loved and cared for her. But Delores, while she loved her parents, always felt a part of her was missing.

"It doesn't seem to matter how much my parents love me—I just can't get over knowing that the woman who gave birth to me didn't want me. I was only a baby. Who doesn't love a baby? I know she was young, but young women raise families all the time. I feel like it was something wrong with me that made her reject me."

Delores suffered the effects of an experience with situational devaluation in response to being given up at birth by her mother. While she feels loved by her adoptive parents, there is a part of her self-worth that was wounded by what she perceived as her birth mother's rejection of her when she was only an infant.

Devaluation also can occur with respect to pervasive conditions such as having membership in a group that is socially stigmatized, ostracized, or marginalized (e.g., racial minorities, females, gays and lesbians). Fifteen-year-old Ben explained:

"I'm afraid to tell anyone I'm gay because I see how people feel about gays. Last week in the locker room I heard a few of the guys talking about a player from the other team who they thought was gay. They said he was a 'fuckin fag' and they ought to 'kick his sissy ass' and 'teach him a few things about being a real man.' That scared me to death. How can I come out when I know it's not just a matter of people calling me names or not wanting to be friends with me? It's a matter of my life."

Ben's plight as a gay youth is representative of many teens across the nation who suffer from pervasive devaluation related to their sexual orientation. As Ben stated, the devaluation he suffers extends from having to listen to anti-gay remarks, to the risk of peer rejection, and even serious threats to his physical safety. The devaluation that Ben experiences as a gay youth forces him to "stay closeted," which means he must endure repeated assumptions of his heterosexuality by friends and family, hide his relationship with his boyfriend, and listen silently when people make cruel and ignorant comments about homosexuality.

Disruption/erosion of community constitutes the second aggravating factor of adolescent violence. Community is an emotional, psychological, and physical phenomenon. It is a place, physical but mostly metaphysical, of rootedness and belonging, where one feels a sense of connection and purpose. The establishment and maintenance of a strong sense of community are necessary preconditions for feeling safe, secure, and connected with others. Adolescents, like their adult counterparts, depend on "community" to derive a sense of identity, rootedness, and positive relations with others. When one's sense of community has been disrupted or eroded, it contributes to a myriad of difficulties. The forces that potentially disrupt community may range from familial issues such as abuse, divorce, separation, and abandonment to broader social issues such as racial, gender, and economic oppression. We have found that there are at least three levels of community that are integral in the lives of adolescents: primary, extended, and cultural (we will describe and discuss each of these levels in greater depth in Chapter 3). When disruption or erosion occurs at two or three of these levels, it greatly exacerbates the risk of violence.

Tonya is a full-blooded Sioux Indian. For generations her ancestors lived in a state of balance with one another and the earth. With the arrival of the white man, all that changed. Tonya's people were subjected to horrific acts of brutality by whites. One way in which white people assaulted many Native American societies was by taking children away from their parents and communities and placing them in boarding schools, where they were "resocialized" to become "good white Christians."

"I remember we were never allowed to talk our language. We couldn't practice any of our traditions or customs that are sacred to our people. If we were caught doing or saying anything Indian, we were severely punished. I missed my parents so much, my whole family. I missed my people and our ways. I cried every night. I kept praying that tomorrow I would be freed and would be able to go home, but tomorrow never came."

Tonya's experience involved the disruption of community at all three levels. She was ripped away from her primary, extended, and cultural communities. Life in the boarding school meant the disruption of community at all three levels not only in the physical sense but also in the existential, metaphysical sense. In the boarding schools, all that Tonya valued as a Native American was devalued. Hence, her experiences reflected the intersection of the disruption of community and devaluation.

Both devaluation and disruption/erosion of community involve some form of "loss." Among teens who turn violent, we have found that their lives tend to be besieged by losses and, most notably, by the *dehumanization of loss*, which is the third aggravating factor. Repeated experiences of unacknowledged and unmourned loss contribute to the dehumanization of loss that is a precursor to violence. It's one thing to lose something that was important to you, but it is far worse when no one in your universe recognizes that you have lost it. The failure to acknowledge another's loss is to deny that person's humanity. Hence, when loss remains unacknowledged, we refer to this as the *dehumanization of loss*, which is the mega-loss. When adolescents, especially those of color, are besieged with unacknowledged, unmourned, and therefore unhealed losses, they are suffering from the dehumanization of loss.

Several months ago we conducted a workshop on loss during which a participant shared an example she had noted with regard to the dehumanization of loss in the lives of children of color.

"I am a teacher in a school where 70% of the children are African American and Hispanic. My husband teaches at a school in a nearby town where only 10% of the children are of color. Three weeks ago, at the school where my husband teaches, a 15-year-old boy, who was white, was shot to death on the playground by another 15-year-old boy, who also was white. The school responded to the event by bringing in a whole team of psychologists, grief counselors, and social workers. They spent almost a week trying to help the kids understand what had happened and providing supportive services. Most of the school attended the funeral, and children wrote poems and stories about the tragic loss of a young life. The thing is, at the school I teach in, we've had four young people die in similar incidents just this past year, and you know what happens? Nothing. They just come in and mop up the blood and we keep right on going, business as usual. I have kids sitting in my room that are obviously suffering from trauma shock, but no one notices, no one cares. If they fall behind academically, or start acting up, we say it's because they aren't smart, don't care about school, or are just plain bad. But they're suffering and the thing is, we don't care about their losses. Because they're kids of color, they must be used to this type of violence—that's the attitude. We don't treat their pain the same as we treat the pain of white children."

As this woman's comments reveal, the children of color in her community and across the country often suffer many painful losses. However, because they are devalued as people of color, their losses are devalued. Their losses, no matter how significant, remain unacknowledged, unmourned, and unhealed. In short, they suffer from the dehumanization of loss.

The phenomenon of *rage* is the final aggravating factor. Rage is the product that emerges from the confluence of devaluation, disruption of community, and the dehumanization of loss. It is a natural and inevitable response to experiences of pain and injustice. When rage is channeled constructively, it can be a positive and transformative force. However, when rage is denied expression or treated as if it is negative, it intensifies and usually culminates in an eruption of violence. In this sense, rage is a mediating variable between the first three factors and violence. The presence of the first three factors gives birth to rage, and depending upon how rage is handled, it may eventually explode into violence.

THE RELATIONSHIP BETWEEN BIOLOGY AND OUR MODEL

Most variables that lead to adolescent violence are reflected in some aspect of our model, but there is one obvious exception: neuropsychiatric and biologically-based factors. Dorothy Lewis, in her landmark 1992 study on the roots of violent behavior, found that violent offenders had higher rates of impulsivity, hyperactivity, attention deficits, and learning disabilities than did non-offenders. Moreover, violent offenders also had histories of prenatal complications and serious injuries and accidents that occurred in early life, more often than was found among non-offenders. These findings point toward a link between biological factors and violence.

According to Karr-Morse and Wiley (1997):

> In order to understand the tide of violent behavior in which America is now submerged, we must look before preadolescence, before grade school, before preschool to the cradle of human formation in the first thirty-three months of life. Those months, including nine months of prenatal development and the first two years after birth (33 months), harbor the seeds of violence for a growing percentage of American children. (p. 9)

Karr-Morse and Wiley paint a compelling picture of the influence that neglect and/or maltreatment have during the 9 months of fetal development and first 24 months after birth. While neither suggests that biologically based factors cause violence, they believe that environmental conditions strongly influence biology during a critical period of development, and the biological alterations that occur in response to environmental shaping predisposes some children more than others to violence later in life. It is here where we see the convergence between biology and our model. As stated by Karr-Morse and Wiley:

> Genes may have a role in shaping later violent behavior, but environmentally altered rather than inherited genes are implicated. In order for those genes to even have an adverse role in later behavior, they must interact with negative factors in the child's environment. For example, during the early critical period of maturation of the brain, prolonged periods of intense stress may actually alter DNA, the building material of the genes. (p. 10)

While biology does influence things such as one's degree of aggressiveness and impulse control, environmental factors play a vital role in shaping biological factors. Fetal alcohol syndrome alters the maturation of infants and places them at an increased risk for developing hyperactivity, attention deficits, aggressiveness, and impulsivity, all of which have been correlated with violence in later life. Moreover, external/environmental factors shape how caretakers (and others as well) respond to a child's biologically based characteristics. If the behavioral effects of fetal alcohol syndrome are such that they engender frustration and rejection from primary caretakers, the young child is now at risk for experiences with devaluation, disruption of community, unacknowledged loss, and rage. This is where we see the convergence of biology and our model. Biologically based risk factors can increase children's vulnerability to developing the four aggravating factors. Hence, biological factors do not de facto mean that a child will become violent later in life. They simply increase the potential risk. According to our work in this area, as long as children have experiences that block the four aggravating factors from developing, the inevitability of violence is thwarted.

OUR AUDIENCE

Our work with violent adolescents has brought us into contact with a variety of professionals, including therapists, teachers, youth workers, probation officers, child welfare advocates, caseworkers, and human service administrators. While all of these professionals think about young people in differing ways, and have different avenues for intervening with troubled teens, there are commonalities that link them all. Most share in common a love and concern for young people. Most have devoted substantial energy toward trying to make connections with youth in need. Many have made personal sacrifices to try to help the most troubled of our teens. Most professionals want the best for kids, but they also have struggled with frustrations when it comes to trying to help. Some of these frustrations range from inadequate social policies, to limited budgets, poorly designed programs, professional burnout, and exhaustion. In the case of violent and aggressive adolescents the frustrations that many professionals share in common tend to be rooted in the absence of a comprehensive model for understanding the factors that contribute to youth violence, coupled with insufficient strategies and resources for addressing the problem.

Our goal in writing this book is to reach out to a range of professionals who may approach their work with violent teens from differing professional angles but who share in common a compassion for kids and a desire to make substantial inroads toward addressing and deterring adolescent violence. At the same time, we also feel a deep commitment to reach out to lay readers as well. We believe that our most effective approach to addressing adolescent violence is through involving adults at all levels. Hence, we wish to engage not only a diverse range of professionals but also nonprofessionals whose lives interface with youth who are at risk of violence. In that vein, we have tried to write in a way that keeps in mind the parent or other concerned adult who is dealing with a young person who is either teetering on the brink or has crossed over into violence.

Clearly we are casting our net broadly, trying to reach out to connect with a diverse readership that interfaces with adolescents in very different ways and on differing levels. As a result, the assumptions we make about the prior knowledge, experience, and agendas of our readers are necessarily broad and fairly general. We assume, for example, that most readers of this book care about young people and are deeply concerned about the violence that is threatening to destroy a generation. We assume that all readers of this book have their own assumptions and ideas about what contributes to adolescent violence and what needs to be done to deal with this problem. Yet, at the same time, we believe that our readers have encountered obstacles and limitations associated with current approaches to addressing this problem, and they are eager for new perspectives and they want to learn innovative intervention strategies. Finally, we assume that most of those who are reading this book have at least one young person in mind whom they are concerned about, are struggling with, and/or feel some sense of anguish over how to reach out and save this person from the clutches of certain doom.

We write with the hope that, through sharing our views of what contributes to adolescent violence, each reader will be able to extract something—whether it's a single insight or a more complex and complete conceptual framework that will assist him or her in understanding this phenomenon. We also write with the ultimate purpose of offering clear-cut practical strategies that most concerned adults, professional or otherwise, can easily employ and that will have some positive effect on ameliorating the danger they foresee or have experienced in relation to the teens with whom they are interacting.

HOW THIS BOOK IS ORGANIZED

After having said much in a general way about the four aggravating factors, we devote the remainder of the first part of this book to examining each one in depth. To bring each of the factors "to life," we offer numerous examples of young people with whom we have interacted. We discuss each factor as an independent concept, but in reality all four are tightly interwoven and shape and inform one another in complex ways.

In the second part of the book we turn to the issue of how to translate the model into action. We present chapters that offer specific practical suggestions for how to address each of the aggravating factors. Our approach here is oriented toward both prevention and intervention. Not surprisingly, we often are asked about adolescents who may have all four aggravating factors present in their lives and yet who have never become violent. Kids like these frequently lead to the question "If this teenager has all four factors in his life, why has he never turned violent?" The answer to this question is integral to a preventative approach to adolescent violence. Among this group of teens, we have found that, in spite of the presence of the four factors, almost all of them have had experiences that counteracted devaluation, restored community, rehumanized loss, and rechanneled rage, which all played a vital role in preventing the trajectory toward violence. Hence, in part two of the book, we present detailed suggestions for how readers can counteract devaluation, restore community, rehumanize loss, and rechannel rage in the lives of adolescents, thereby intervening to disrupt current violence and preventing future violence from occurring.

CHAPTER 2

• • • • • • •

Devaluation

Timothy Ryan was 15 when he and a pair of friends attacked a boy and a girl who were walking home from a movie together. They beat the couple so badly that they both had to be hospitalized. They raped the girl. A witness who saw them running from the scene identified the boys, and they were arrested hours later. When questioned by the police, Timothy admitted his involvement without remorse, proclaiming, "I told him not to mess with me, but he didn't listen. He got what was coming to him. And although that little rich bitch always acted like she thought she was better than everyone else, I didn't touch her."

Kate and Shaun Ryan sat before us looking shell-shocked. They knew their son had done some troubling things before this, like attacking his younger brother and punching a hole in a bedroom door. But they never could have imagined that their son could go this far. Kate, seemingly oblivious to our presence, wondered aloud but to herself:

"What happened to the innocent boy I used to bake chocolate chip cookies for? I can still see him smiling, his eyes twinkling as he grabbed two cookies at once, smearing chocolate everywhere. I can still hear him asking for 'just one, Mommy ... please, Mommy.' "

That was how she remembered him; he was eager, hungry to taste the sweetness of life, and unfettered by his slightly clumsy demeanor.

Where was that child now? What had happened since then to transform Timothy into such a bitter, cynical, angry young teenager?

The Ryans' questions are not unlike those that parents and other concerned adults all across this nation are asking in response to the disturbing numbers of once seemingly "normal, happy" children who have mutated into cold, heartless adolescent aggressors. One of the things that makes Timothy's case compelling is the fact that prior to his violent attack on the couple there was little on the surface that revealed the trauma and unrest that were dwelling within the Ryan household. Several members of the community expressed shock and disbelief when they learned of Timothy's violence because when they looked at him they saw a quiet, intelligent boy from a "normal family."

When we look beyond the surface and the stereotypes about "normal" and "ideal," we quickly find that among kids who become violent there are several common features they all share. The first of these involves devaluation, which is a process that strips a person or a group of dignity and a sense of worth. Devaluation is like an untreated cancer that attacks deep inside one's core. It slowly eats away at one's sense of self-esteem, and often does so unbeknownst to the affected individual or group. All of us have experiences with devaluation at some point in our lives. What is most important to bear in mind with adolescents who become violent is that, in addition to suffering from multiple experiences with devaluation, even more significantly the emotional wounds inflicted by devaluation go largely untreated and unhealed, which has a crippling emotional effect.

There are two types of devaluation: situational and societal. Situational devaluation occurs when the source of the devaluation is limited to a specific time and place. It is idiosyncratic in nature and involves any circumstance or event that assaults the dignity of those affected. Situational devaluation is distinguishable from societal devaluation, which refers to the degradation that an individual or group experiences as a result of having membership in a group that is marginalized by or within society. Societal devaluation is inextricably tied to broader social forces such as class, gender, race, and sexual orientation. Given our conceptualization of devaluation, it is highly conceivable that one individual could simultaneously suffer from both situational and societal devaluation. While one could certainly argue that devaluation is devaluation, we believe the distinctions that we have drawn are necessary because they have strong implications for how we work with violent and aggressive youth.

SITUATIONAL DEVALUATION

The factors associated with situational devaluation can range from experiences with incessant childhood rejection to learning disabilities. The forces that contribute to situational devaluation are virtually countless and quite varied. They often cover a wide range of experiences that are not always predictable or easy to discern. After years of working with troubled youth, we have found that there are several strains of situational devaluation that are most common among adolescents who have some propensity toward violence and aggression. We have found evidence of abandonment, abuse, and social ostracism among the overwhelming number of violent youth with whom we have worked. Because abandonment, abuse, and social ostracism are repeatedly associated with situational devaluation and ultimately violence, we want to provide a closer look at these concepts.

Abandonment

Timothy Ryan, in many respects, was a textbook example of devaluation associated with abandonment and abuse. When we started our work with the Ryan family, we tried to identify where, in his life, Timothy might have encountered devaluation. This was no easy task. Timothy was committed to not talking to us during the first few weeks of therapy, and his parents, while willing to talk, had great difficulty doing so about anything that they feared might portray them as bad parents.

"We've been good parents," Shaun exclaimed. "We set limits for our kids. We don't allow any crazy stuff. We spend time with the kids. Let's put it this way: I see my kids more than my dad ever saw me or my brothers."

Kate agreed with her husband. "We tried to teach the kids morals. I take them to church every week. Timothy and Robert are very involved with our church. We did everything we could think of. What more could we have done as parents?"

Like many parents, the Ryans were focused on all the things they had done right. It was too painful for them to see the things that had happened that might have hurt their son, even though they never wanted to hurt him—like the fact that the Ryan's had spent the first few years of their marriage arguing constantly. When Timothy was 5, his parents had a fight that was so bitter his father left for 6 months. Although his parents later reconciled, little Timothy was left carrying the scars of his parents' early marital strife. As we eventually discovered after months of therapy, when Shaun left the family, Timothy felt abandoned and blamed himself for his father's departure. This experience, at such a young vulnerable age, deeply wounded Timothy and was a source of pain and shame—a form of situational devaluation that continued to haunt him 10 years later.

When this traumatic episode that had occurred early in the Ryans' marriage finally came to light, both parents dismissed it as "something from the past." It was difficult for them to believe that something that had happened so long ago could have had any impact on Timothy's present troubles. They had difficulty relating to how Timothy might have perceived things as a little boy. When we suggested that Timothy felt abandoned by his father when he was 5 and blamed himself, Shaun lashed back: "That's ridiculous. I never abandoned my family. We just needed space apart, and it actually helped. It had nothing to do with Timothy. Besides, that was 10 years ago."

Unfortunately, it was hard for Shaun to put himself into the mind of a 5-year-old and imagine how things must have seemed from Timothy's perspective. Shaun found it difficult to acknowledge the deep insecurities that Timothy suffered from as a result of his earlier childhood experiences. Acknowledging that his decision to leave Timothy (and the family) at such an early age could have possibly left his son feeling abandoned was simply too painful for Shaun. It stirred up feelings of guilt and failure.

It's important to stress that this experience alone did not lead to Timothy's violence, but it played a role. It was one of the threads that had been woven into his evolving psychosocial tapestry. It has been our clinical experience that abandonment is difficult to contend with at any age. However, it is particularly challenging when it occurs in childhood. There probably is no other human experience that confirms for a child his or her lack of worth in the way that abandonment does. It probably sounds ludicrous and disingenuous to discuss abandonment and abuse in terms of which is actually worse, since both are exceedingly harmful. However, we believe that, while both can be painfully harmful, abandonment is usually more devastating. The deep feeling of personal rejection that usually accompanies abandonment provides the foundation for devaluation and ultimately the assault on one's sense of personhood, dignity, and self-respect. Abuse, even in its most horrific forms, usually does not leave most children feeling unloved. Most abused children are left with very ambivalent and complex feelings about themselves and those who have abused them, especially if it has been a parental figure. It is common for the abandoned child to typically think of him- or herself as unworthy and unlovable, while the abused child frequently thinks of him- or herself as bad.

Abuse

Abuse is another common factor associated with situational devaluation in the lives of young people. Victims of abuse often blame themselves for their victimization. All too often, they conclude that it was some defect of theirs that invited the maltreatment. Deep within, most abused kids believe either that they are inherently unworthy of love and affirmation by their parents and/or caretakers or that the abusive behavior is their parents' way of demonstrating love. In either case, the result is usually the same: devaluation.

With time and patience the Ryans began to trust us a little more, and gradually they began to disclose more about their family. In particular, we found out that when Timothy was very young, his father was often verbally and physically abusive toward him. After the Ryans reconciled, Shaun learned to manage his behavior and feelings more effectively, but Timothy's scars remained unhealed. Because Timothy was so young when the abuse occurred, he was virtually defenseless against the barrage of critical, contemptuous, condemning messages he received from his father. Each angry word, raised voice, and irritable expression was evidence to the young Timothy that he was unloved and unwanted by his father. Moreover, each time Shaun Ryan slapped Timothy's cheek, swatted the back of his head, or pounded his fist into his back, he was wielding a blow against the very core of his son's fragile sense of self. These experiences were a form of situational devaluation. They were wounding events that had occurred in the past, and it didn't matter that Shaun no longer did these things. Because the wounds had never been treated or healed, they continued to fester within Timothy, crippling some piece of his spirit.

Abused children and adolescents often internalize intense feelings of shame and humiliation. Because they believe their own deficiencies are the basis for the abuse, they interpret it as a stain on their sense of dignity and pride. Abused kids will often attempt to keep the abuse hidden from view for fear that if others knew it would expose something "bad" about themselves. In this way, abused kids suffer from both the actual pain involved in the abuse and the emotional pain that lasts long after the physical wounds have healed. The emotional wounds are rooted in a belief that the abuse is proof that one is a bad, maybe unlovable, person. The feeling of "badness" is linked to a deep sense of shame that accompanies doubts about one's self-worth and value as a human being. We especially observe this among children and adolescents who are victims of sexual abuse. The general stigma attached to sex intensifies the feelings of shame and lack of worth that victims of sexual abuse often experience. Long after the abuse is over and the physical scars have disappeared from view, the emotional damage of abuse and the sense of devaluation it breeds, if untreated and unhealed, can last a lifetime.

In Timothy's case, his experiences with situational devaluation profoundly deformed his sense of self. Long after the bruises on his arms and back had healed, the bruises on his fragile self-esteem remained painfully ripe. No further evidence is needed of Timothy's self-hate than the extreme acts of violence toward those whom he viewed as weaker and more helpless. His actions revealed the part of his psyche that identified with feeling weak and helpless; he hated that feeling within himself so intensely that he had to destroy it any cost. With each assault he wielded upon someone of a weaker stature, it was as if he were punishing himself for his own weakness and helplessness in the face of a more powerful aggressive force. It was as if he were trying to annihilate the very weaknesses and helplessness within himself that had made him vulnerable in the past. In fact, in a therapy session with Timothy and his parents, his mother painfully said, "I don't understand how someone can be begging you to stop hurting them, and you just don't stop." Timothy responded by saying, "If they gotta beg, they don't deserve for it to stop."

Timothy's comment again revealed the contempt he held for any sign of vulnerability, stemming from the resentment he felt toward his own vulnerability and the ways it had made him a target for abuse. For Timothy, his vulnerability made him feel "less than," which is at the heart of experiences with devaluation. Those who are devalued struggle incessantly with feeling "less than." And, as we learned more about Timothy, the more apparent it became that his experiences with situational devaluation were inextricably linked to a profound sense of feeling "less than," which played a salient role in his violence toward others.

Divorce

For many young people divorce is another common factor associated with situational devaluation. It is not our view nor has it been our experience that divorce de facto translates into devaluation. In fact, we have seen repeatedly that it is the quality of the experience that ultimately dictates the impact that it has on the life of the child. When divorce is carried out in a way that keeps the child's needs and welfare in the forefront of the experience, devaluation is averted. However, when the child, on the other hand, is caught in the crossfire of the parents' bitter acrimony, devaluation is very likely. Anisha Jenkins's parents divorced when she was only 4 years old. Her father left her mother to marry another woman. The divorce was brimming with bitterness and pain. Anisha's mother felt profoundly rejected and betrayed by her husband. The divorce devastated her emotionally and severely impaired her financially. Although 12 years had passed, she still felt extreme rage toward her ex-husband and his second wife. She still bad-mouthed him anytime his name entered the conversation. When Anisha wanted to buy a prom dress or asked for money to go on a senior class trip to Washington, DC, her mother's reply was always some version of the following: "Ask your no-good, playboy, rich father. Thanks to him I can't afford to give you these things."

During the same 12 years, Anisha's father was also still stuck in feelings of anger and contempt toward his former wife. He still referred to her as "a selfish, vindictive woman who would have sucked all the life out of me if I had stayed with her." Twelve years after the divorce, when Anisha came to her father for money for her prom dress, he told her, "If your mother managed her finances better, you wouldn't have to come to me for this." As a result, Anisha had spent the last 12 years of her life trapped between hostile parents who had been unable to resolve their feelings of bitterness, contempt, and pain. Unfortunately, each time one of them fired a missile at the other, Anisha was wounded by the resulting explosion.

Sitting in our office looking small and helpless with tears streaming quietly down her face, Anisha told us she would do anything to stop her parents from hating each other. She complained that their hatred for each other made it impossible for them to love her or for her to feel close to either one of them. Her voice was filled with anguished yearning. At the age of 4 she had lived through ground zero of her parent's nuclear explosion—their divorce.

Divorces that are characterized by high doses of resentment, contempt, and bitterness tend to be devaluing to all concerned. If friends and family perceive the divorce as a shameful event, and if one or both partners fail to receive support or compassion from loved ones, the divorce can be extremely devaluing. Moreover, when a divorcing couple fails to find a way to retain their parental relationship in the midst of severing their marital relationship, divorce can be extremely disruptive to children and adolescents. These types of divorce, from a child's perspective, are tantamount to abandonment. We routinely hear kids say:

- "I was afraid I would never see my mother or father again—like maybe they didn't love me anymore."
- "I felt like it was my fault that my parents got a divorce. Maybe if I had been better, this never would have happened."
- "My family is gone now. Now that my parents are getting a divorce, I won't have a family anymore."

Each of these comments is a typical response from kids of divorcing parents, especially when the parents do not find healthy ways of negotiating the experience. Each of these common responses is also indicative of devaluation. In these scenarios, the kids in question relate to their parents' divorce by seeing it as something that reflects negatively upon them. They view the divorce as evidence of their inherent deficiencies, and therefore they hold themselves responsible for the breakup. These comments also reveal the sense of losing something that was valuable and, hence, of feeling less valuable themselves. In other words, many kids typically interpret divorce to mean that they no longer have a whole family, which becomes equated with not being a whole person. In this way, for some kids, the divorce constitutes a fracturing of their families—and therefore of themselves—making them "less than." This is the epitome of devaluation.

Peer Rejection: Kids Who Are Outcasts

In some instances the roots of situational devaluation are tied to something that is specific to an individual. We commonly see this with kids who are labeled and treated as outcasts by their peers because they aren't attractive enough, athletic enough, charismatic enough, or because they are too fat or too skinny, too brainy, or, as one teen told us, "just plain weird." For kids like these, social ostracism is the consequence. While all people crave affirmation to some degree, this need is especially intense for adolescents. Few adults reading this will have to stretch their imagination to understand the awkwardness and uncertainty that haunts most adolescents. No matter what our contemporary experiences are, each of us has advanced through this difficult period of development, and while the transition was smoother for some than for others, it is probably safe to say that all of us had at least some encounter with pangs of insecurity, fears of rejection, and anxiety about wanting to "fit in" and be accepted. For kids "who don't fit in" in the ways that matter to prevailing peer norms, their fate as outcasts can be worse than death.

Situational devaluation as "outcasts" was evident in the lives of Eric Harris and Dylan Klebold, the infamous teenaged pair who murdered 12 of their fellow students and a teacher during a shooting rampage in April 1999 at Columbine High School in Litttleton, Colorado. As criminologists, sociologists, and mental health experts began to piece together clues about the lives of both boys, what eventually emerged were portraits of two teenagers who felt profoundly devalued by their peers. They were outcasts, scorned and rejected by their contemporaries. In typical teen fashion, the two boys did not let their feelings of rejection, hurt, and shame show outwardly. They mostly kept their pain hidden from view, buried beneath the black trench coats they wore menacingly to school. Yet, in retrospect, it requires little effort to see the deep-seated feelings of isolation, alienation, and rejection that both boys felt in relation to their peers. In a word, they suffered from devaluation.

Eric and Dylan had compiled a "hit list" of students they intended to target during their reign of terror. These were kids who had been the most rejecting and scornful toward them. In their mind's eye, these other kids were perpetrators, and they were victims—victims who had developed a plot to righteously reclaim their dignity and avenge their battered sense of honor. Obviously, their plan was grossly twisted and lacking in perspective. And yet, the extreme nature of their actions provides a clue about how the world looked inside the borders of their minds. For Eric and Dylan, the scorn and rejection they felt from peers was gargantuan. The injustices they experienced at the hands of some of their schoolmates were a matter of "life and death"a matter so severe that the only way they thought they could balance the scales of justice was by taking the lives of (as it turned out) 13 people. One can only imagine how intensely these two boys must have felt persecuted, rejected, and utterly devalued to devise a retaliatory plan of such extreme destructiveness.

In addition to revealing how deeply devalued by their peers Eric and Dylan felt, the diaries, letters, and videotapes they left behind demonstrate how firmly resolved they were about their own deaths. They were willing to die to save their dignity. They stated explicitly that they never planned to survive their attack upon the school. They were clear that, by seeking retribution for the crimes they believed had been committed against them, they would have to sacrifice their own lives. From their perspective, they were going to die for the sake of their dignity, which was preferable to living with the dishonor and disgrace that came with their status as outcasts. In this way, Eric and Dylan were like many of the urban, mostly African American and Latino, adolescents we work with from poor, gang-infested communities.

Like Eric and Dylan, many urban poor, minority teens are driven by a similar mantra: "death before dis" ("dis" being an abbreviated form for "disrespect"). While Eric and Dylan were responding to situational devaluation related to being personally rejected by their community of peers, many adolescents of color residing within inner cities are subjected to societal devaluation (we will say more about this in the following section) associated with their intersecting racial and class identities. We have lost count of the number of times we have heard a Latino or African American youth defiantly assert that he hit (or worse) another youth for "dissing" him. Moreover, the nature of the "dis" is often something that seems benign to those who are not young, poor, and a person of color. For example, Steve, a 15-year-old male whose mother was Puerto Rican and father was African American, proudly described to us how he "busted that doughboys butt for steppin' on my sneaks." He went on to explain that by stepping on Steve's sneakers—and worse, by not expressing extreme contrition—this other boy was essentially stepping on Steve's honor.

Whenever he recounts this story to adults, they often become reactive to Steve. They cannot understand how such a minor infraction could justify such an extreme act of aggression. But what typically gets missed is that Steve and those like him live in a world where the opportunities for validation and respect are amazingly sparse, and almost every aspect of their identities and lives is denigrated. In their world, respect is a rare commodity of such value that many are willing to kill or die to obtain it.

EXPERIENCES WITH SITUATIONAL DEVALUATION AND THE WOUNDS OF DEVALUATION

As stated earlier, there is an important distinction between the actual experience that has an initial impact in the moment, on the one hand, and the emotional–psychological wounds that result, which if untreated and unhealed, can persist and remain a source of pain and shame long after the actual event has passed. Ravaged by the wounds of the actual divorce with all the cruel words, hateful acts, and vicious maneuvers, Anisha Jenkins might have been able to begin to heal over time except that the fallout from the bitter and contentious separation had never been addressed. The toxic emotional energy that had been generated had never dissipated. As a result, Anisha grew up watching episodes of the *Cosby Show*, fantasizing that the Huxtables were her family. She looked at her friends with envy and tried to imagine what it would be like "to grow up in a normal family." After her parents got embroiled in a screaming match at one of her soccer games when she was 9, Anisha spent endless hours carefully planning the exact school events and soccer games she would invite each of her parents to attend. She never wanted them together in public again—the risk of personal humiliation was just too high. She still wasn't sure how she would handle her graduation, as this was one thing that she still had not worked out in her plan.

When Shaun Ryan left his family, this was a devaluing event in Timothy's life. The event was time-limited, lasting for just 6 months. But Timothy suffered deep emotional and psychological wounds from the event, which he perceived as abandonment. Additionally, Shaun's physical and verbal abusiveness with Timothy, while it only occurred during his early childhood, left emotional and psychological wounds that persisted long after the actual events had passed. Years later, Timothy was still suffering from devaluation rooted in the time when his father was gone, as well as the times when his father was abusively present.

According to Timothy, several weeks after his father left he was taunted by a neighborhood boy who was a few years older. "He told me I didn't have anyone to stick up for me now that my father was gone. I told him my father would be back, and he said it wasn't true. He said my father didn't want me." Although Timothy wore a stoic expression while recounting this experience, the way he suddenly began to swivel his chair alerted us to the underlying emotional intensity he felt many years following that difficult period in his life. Even though his father returned after 6 months and his parents reconciled, Timothy continued to bear the pain of the wound that had been inflicted.

Moreover, imagine the dilemmas Shaun's return created for Timothy when his father beat him with his words and his fists. Whatever relief Timothy felt upon having his father back home inevitably was tempered by the pain of his father's abusiveness. And while the abuse eventually stopped, the adverse effects of these experiences with situational devaluation persisted long after. The same was true for Anisha with respect to her parent's divorce. While the divorce was a time-limited event, the devaluation it generated persisted long after the experience because the wounds inflicted by it were never addressed or ultimately healed. Twelve years after her parents' divorce, Anisha was still struggling with the pain and shame of the devaluation that this event had triggered all those years ago.

THE ALL-CONSUMING CONCERN WITH RESPECT

To be devalued is to be disrespected. One of the central features of those who have been devalued is that they suffer from an exaggerated, all-consuming concern with obtaining respect. Ironically, perpetual efforts to obtain respect often becloud the devaluation that underpins the need for respect. When all of one's energy becomes focused around respect, it is easy for those around to lose sight of the devaluation that drives the need for the respect in the first place. In particular, the ways in which many adolescents strive to obtain respect distracts others from appreciating the underlying devaluation that resides at the heart of their unrelenting quest for respect. Hence, the devaluation that generates the need for respect is obscured by attitude and behaviors associated with the all-consuming quest to gain respect. For example, when one kid shoots another kid who "dissed" him, it is easy to overlook the role that devaluation played in this lethal pursuit for respect.

Respect and the phenomenon of "being dissed" are often at the center of much of our work with schools. We have seen far too much violence, death, and destruction spearheaded by the all consuming concern with respect. We have seen the multitudinous ways in which it can shape every aspect of young peoples' lives while simultaneously remaining invisible to the naked eye. When we consult with teachers and counselors about the relationship between devaluation and respect, we often are posed with the challenge: "It's funny that you would talk about these kids needing respect so much because they are the ones who are the most disrespectful." This is an honest, heartfelt assessment that rarely surprises us. It is entirely reasonable and predictable that the youth who have been the most devalued (and probably disrespected) will also be those who are the most disrespectful. From their perspective, respect is to be "gotten" by any means necessary. Through the eyes of devalued youth, "respect" earned disrespectfully is worthy of respect nonetheless. Their need for respect, and the means of achieving it, is often buried under layers of adolescent bravado. Neither the adolescents nor many of the adults working with them are consciously aware that their behavior is so heavily driven by the connections between devaluation and desire for respect. The adolescents are too often distracted by their "the end justifies the means" philosophy, while most adults get trapped into focusing on the bad, or antisocial, behavior. In both cases, devaluation and the all-consuming concern with respect are overlooked.

Eric Harris and Dylan Klebold were obsessed with respect and willing to die for it. Timothy Ryan was obsessed with respect. After the incident where he beat another boy unmercifully he stated, "I needed to teach him what respect is. He used to think he was all that . . . being all flashy and shit . . . Well, I showed him. . . I'm no punk. He may have some cash but that couldn't save his ass . . . I beat the mothafucker and I would do it again."

It's easy to get distracted by Timothy's belief that violence is the way to solve his problems. Certainly we wished that he had chosen to solve his problems in another way, but we also could see that underneath the bravado was a boy who felt very badly about himself for many reasons. The issue of money and class clearly underpinned Timothy's aggression. His reference to the other boy thinking he was better because he had more money exposed the ways in which Timothy struggled with devaluation related to his working-class status and his family's limited economic resources. To Timothy, all of this translated into an issue of respect. Respect is a rare commodity that is highly valued and difficult to secure for those who have suffered from high doses of devaluation. Those who feel devalued and therefore disrespected will go to almost any length to "take" that which they feel they deserve.

Timothy clearly struggled with not feeling respected. He was consumed with his mission to seek out and, if need be, take respect in whatever way he deemed necessary. This dynamic has been true of virtually every adolescent we have worked with where violence and aggression have been major difficulties. Like so many of his adolescent counterparts, when Timothy felt disrespected, his options for responding were far too limited. Unfortunately, his seemingly rigid and impulsive actions seldom provided a complete portrait of Timothy. Although he always turned to violence as his first, second, third, and final options, what few people ever saw were the painful emotional wounds that his bravado disguised.

Much of our discussion about Timothy has been devoted to an examination of how situational devaluation played such a huge role in his life. We have said very little up to this point about the ways in which societal devaluation also contributed heavily to his ongoing struggles with violence and aggression. We believe that, even if Timothy's relationship with his father had been profoundly different, devaluation would have remained a manifest part of his life experience because of his working-class status, that is, he also experienced devaluation at the societal level.

SOCIETAL DEVALUATION

Whereas situational devaluation is confined to a specific time and place or an experience that is unique to an individual, societal devaluation involves a generalized sense of being dehumanized because of one's membership in a socially stigmatized and depreciated group. Adolescents who are members of socially marginalized groups (e.g., those who are poor or working-class, youth of color, girls, gays or lesbians) are encumbered by a sense of devaluation within themselves at all times.

Youth of Color

A few years ago we interviewed a young African American male named Carter who lived in an economically depressed community. He was talking about how the city was building another prison only a few blocks from his neighborhood. In fact, he could view the rear of the prison grounds from his bedroom window. To Carter, the prison was a symbol of how little the city and society at large cared about him and those like him. He explained:

"When we see that prison, we know it's meant for us. We know they put it here because they want us to know it's for us. Whenever we see it there, we know this society don't care nothing about us. They just want to lock us all up, because they think we are just a bunch of criminals. That's what they see when they look at a young black man. So, if that's how they feel about us, what's the point? We might as well just get high and go out and shoot a nigger. No one expects anything different from us, anyway. They already have our cells ready for us, so what the hell."

As Carter's haunting words depict, he was suffering from the pain of societal devaluation in relation to his identity as a young black (poor) male.

Living within a society that is organized on the basis of a skin color hierarchy creates a complex set of challenges for adolescents of color. While many teens have insecurities about feeling as though they don't fit in, these feelings often are intensified for kids of color, who receive powerful rejecting messages on the basis of their race and skin color. All around them they are exposed to messages that suggest beauty is defined by white skin, blue eyes, thin lips, and a small pointy nose. They are consistently bombarded with messages that defile and devalue anything that is dark and/or associated with negroid features. Because of the pervasiveness of the social programming that occurs with respect to the race/skin color hierarchy, most kids of color cannot graduate from adolescence without having internalized some of the seeds of self-hate. This is true for boys as well as girls.

Jory and Ron were best friends. They had grown up together and were more like brothers than friends. Both were African American males, but Ron was dark-skinned and Jory was light-skinned. While they both shared membership in a socially devalued group, their experiences with devaluation varied in relation to their complexions. According to Ron:

"It makes me so mad how girls always prefer Jory 'cause he's the lighter one. They are always saying how cute and fine he is and how he has nice hair and pretty eyes. It gets to me. It's to the point that I hate looking in the mirror, and I resent this."

According to Jory:

"In America people like what's white . . . or light. The truth is that girls usually like me more 'cause I'm light and I have good hair. I know it bothers Ron . . . and like once he even told me that I think I'm better 'cause I'm light. It's not true, but I can see why he feels that way."

The pain that Ron experienced was directly related to his devaluation as a dark-skinned black person. As a result, he had internalized rejecting messages that were the basis for profound psychic, social, and spiritual pain and hardship. These messages are even more devastating for girls of color, who not only have to deal with race but with gender as well. For girls of color, these dynamics are intensified by the fact that such a large aspect of female identity is tied to physical beauty. We will say more about this in the following section.

Girls

Most girls experience societal devaluation on the basis of their gender. The journey from girlhood toward womanhood involves the struggle to achieve a narrowly defined standard of physical beauty and a disposition toward males that can be characterized simply as "ready and willing to serve." The transition from girlhood into womanhood involves the creation of a sexual object. Yet, paradoxically, the very sexuality that is a girl's passport to womanhood is also the basis of her inevitable defamation and shame. While most girls are eager to "become a woman," interactions with family, friends, teachers, coaches, and the broader culture all teach girls that to do so they must acquire a necessary but highly sinful sexuality. It is this sexuality that will offer the promise of status, validation, and self-worth, but will ultimately deliver, for the majority of girls at least, a strong, disorienting dose of devaluation.

Most boys receive messages that suggest their blossoming sexuality is a source of pride—a vigorous, exquisite, healthy need that should be honored, catered to, and nurtured. In contrast, most girls receive messages that suggest their emerging sexuality is either a passive, barely perceptible flicker unworthy of meaningful consideration or an uncontrollable, vulgar, sinful force that must be curbed, controlled, and contained. Simply stated, girls learn that their emerging sexuality is something to be regarded with shame. Author Naomi Wolf (1997) has captured powerfully the devaluation that girls are subjected to with respect to female sexuality.

> Every day, one of us adolescent girls might hear in conversation in the schoolyard, or on the street, these words: "cunt," "fuck," "pussy," "whore," "bitch," and of course "slut." We shrugged them off again and again but always felt as if a small stain from them clung to us, a show, as Lawrence put it, of dirt. Of course we knew the words were about us, our bodies, our wishes. If we consider the slang terms that describe female

> sexual anatomy, the veil of ugliness through which our culture sees
> women's sexuality is all too obvious. Many have noted that the words
> tend to connote, at their worst, wounds; at best, receptacles. Not one
> slang sexual term—or formal term, for that matter—about women that
> we girls heard encoded the idea of value or preciousness. (p. 182)

As girls journey toward womanhood, they are exposed to a multi-
plicity of messages that convey a profound disrespect for femaleness
in general, and female sexuality more specifically. At best, girls experience their developing bodies as a joke, a source of crude locker room
humor. At worst, they experience their bodies as a license for others
(specifically males) to abuse, exploit, and violate them. Their emerging sexual desire is also a source of profound devaluation. While boys
are affirmed for experiencing their budding sexual needs, girls are
shamed for feeling—let alone, for acting upon—their sexual needs. As
a result, many girls develop protective mechanisms that involve curb-
ing and controlling their sexuality, in some cases, denying it altogether, both to others and to themselves. Girls who do not learn how
to constrain their sexuality are punished in the harshest of ways. They
are targeted for a type of devaluation that transcends the generalized
devaluation that affects all girls. These are the girls who are labeled as
sluts.

As Wolf pointed out, the badness in all girls—their sexuality—
makes all girls "sluts." But only a segment of the population of girls
directly incurs the humiliation of being publicly branded a slut. These
girls become symbolic manifestations of the badness that belongs to
all girls. As such, they carry a disproportionate piece of the burden of
shame that is associated with female sexuality in general.

The rules regarding who is singled out to carry the burden of the
slut label, while arbitrary in one sense, are also mediated by informants such as race and class. Wolf (1997) described a girlhood friend,
Dinah, who lost the maddening game of musical chairs. Dinah was no
more sexually active—and maybe was less so—than Wolf and her
other friends. But because she was female, had developed large breasts
at a young age, walked with her head held high, and was poor, she was
labeled a slut. "Class had declared Dinah a slut by fourteen, while she
was still technically a virgin. It kept her there and kept me and my
other little middle-class friends, who were wilder than she was, just
on the right side of safe" (p. 71).

Dinah's story involved interlocking rings of devaluation. She was
devalued on the basis of several factors—class, gender, physique,
attitude—each of which interacted with and informed the others in a

complex manner. It was each of these, separately, and in terms of how they all fit together that defiled Dinah. It was the fact that she had the nerve to be a poor girl with a voluptuous body who didn't apologize for any of it. One of the most interesting aspects of Dinah's story involved the way that she walked with her head held high, which most likely was both a response to her devaluation (e.g., "If you don't respect me, then screw you. I'll hold my head high to spite you for your low opinion of me") as well as a contributing factor (e.g., she was punished for having the nerve to hold her head high as a poor girl with big breasts).

In spite of the defiant posture Dinah assumed in the face of her devaluation, over time, she began to show signs of weariness. The strain of devaluation left a mark on her. As reported by Wolf:

> Her clothes tighter and her makeup heavier than ever, Dinah still seemed proud and she still carried herself with that head-held-high, fuck-you regalness. . . . But I could see that something was getting worn down in her. By the time we started high school, there were always dark circles under her eyes. She seemed to me to look fatigued from the effort it all took. (p. 71)

For girls of color, the interaction between gender and race makes for an even more complex experience in terms of devaluation. In U.S. culture, sexuality and physical beauty constitute the defining features of female worth. Yet, we also impose narrowly defined standards of beauty that are blatantly racist. Hence, for a female to be deemed beautiful and desirable in mainstream U.S. society, she must be white, thin, with large breasts and a flat stomach, and ideally with silky blond hair, blue eyes, and narrow, angular facial features. This is the archetypal American beauty. Certainly this norm means that most American females, by virtue of body size alone, do not measure up to the standard. But more poignantly, it means that virtually no female of color can ever fulfill this standard by virtue of her skin color. Girls of color are also less likely than their white counterparts to measure up to the ideal by virtue of their more typical heavier figures, the thickness of their hair texture, and the shape of facial features.

Poor and Working-Class Youth

One of the great American myths is of the classless society. In reality, class is a powerful shaper of social reality. While the indicators of class are often subtle, and rarely recognized consciously or named overtly, they organize human relationships in powerful ways. One of the inevitable consequences of living in a class-based society is that attributions about the moral, intellectual, and social worth of individuals and families are made on the basis of class. For those who are members of the middle and upper classes, assumptions of innate value and decency are made. Conversely, the lower-income and working classes of society are often equated with deficiency and worthlessness. I (KVH) will never forget when I was the plaintiff in a personal injury case. The day before we were to appear in court I was reviewing various aspects of the case with my attorney. At the time I was wearing what I refer to as my "comfortable clothes." Needless to say, the wear and tear was showing. These clothes looked as if I had owned them for most of my life. Toward the end of our conversation my attorney said, "I don't suppose I need to tell you that what you wear tomorrow is important. I would stay away from anything like what you have on now. Try one of your most expensive suits instead." I was intrigued by his statement.

"I would think it would be a mistake to go in there tomorrow looking as if I am well-off. Won't that undermine the jury's sympathy for me? Won't they say that I look like I'm doing okay already, and use that as a rationale to vote against me?"

I'll never forget my attorney's response. He explained, "What you're saying makes sense only if you're thinking in terms of justice. But this isn't a just world, professor. If you go into court tomorrow looking like you're poor, the jury will give you what they think you're worth—nothing."

These words have haunted me ever since because I know that they reflect a cold truth. The members of the jury, like all of us, would draw certain class-based conclusions about who I was as a person, and these would inform their decision.

While his reference to the jury pertained to the 12 men and women who would be deciding my case, in fact, the jury is an excellent metaphor for all of us as members of this society. To some degree, we all sit in judgment, drawing conclusions about one another's character and worth based on a variety of factors, not the least of which is class. Most often, our attention to class, and the ways in which it shapes our perceptions and behaviors, occurs outside of our awareness. But whether we are aware of it or not, "the facts" often have little to do with the class-based judgments we pass. We live in a society that confuses class with character. So, if the jury members perceived me as poor, they would have less respect and consideration for me as a human being. I would become "less than" in their eyes, and as a result, they would give me less. On the other hand, if they viewed me as middle- to upper-class, they would unconsciously translate my socioeconomic worth into my worth as a person. Because they would conclude I was more of a human being, they would be more inclined to grant me more.

Several years ago we were conducting an in-service training workshop with the faculty of a law school at a large university. I (TAL) had forgotten we had the training that day, and as a result I did not dress accordingly. I wore slacks and a sweater that were visibly of a low quality. Nonetheless, I didn't think any more about this until days later when speaking with a colleague who was friendly with a woman on the law school faculty who had participated in the training. As my colleague related to me, her friend reported to her that the training was useful, but she was especially surprised by me. Apparently, upon seeing me for the first time, this woman's first impression was that she "didn't expect much." She was shocked once we actually got started and the training developed, because she actually found me "to be surprisingly assertive, poised, and competent." When my colleague inquired about what had led to her initial erroneous impression of me, the woman replied: "I don't exactly know. Some of it was probably how she was dressed. She just looked like she was probably poor."

This woman's assumptions are revealing in several ways. First, there is the issue regarding the types of markers she used to determine my class status. Somehow, just by looking at me, she saw something that led her to make conclusions about my class status, and in particular, that I was poor. While I do not know exactly what led to that conclusion, I strongly suspect that how I was dressed had much to do with her assumption. The second issue involves the leap she made from deducing I was poor, to not expecting very much from me. For this woman, poor people are less competent and less worthy of being given the benefit of the doubt.

The assumptions this faculty member made were powerful, and most likely outside of her consciousness, which is the case with most of us. But imagine how these assumptions and her lack of self-awareness might have affected her role as a faculty member interacting with students. When meeting with students whose clothes imply they are poor, it seems reasonable to wonder if she might expect less from these students, and perhaps even grade their assignments more (or possibly less) stringently than their assumed to be middle- to upper-class counterparts. The really complicated aspect of this is that class-based assumptions are rarely acknowledged and openly discussed. Consequently, some of her students, who may have felt subtly devalued or slighted in their interactions with her, would never have had the benefit of knowing the influence that class biases had had. Just imagine how many times every day little offenses like these probably occur, with little or no opportunity for those who are assaulted to seek any confirmation that an assault has occurred, let alone an opportunity for redress.

Ironically, had I grown up poor, I probably would never have allowed myself to leave my apartment dressed as I was on the day of the law school training. The devaluation that poor and working-class people feel propels many to engage in compensatory behaviors designed to challenge perceptions of their economic poverty and the devaluation that accompanies these. It never ceases to amaze us how many poor teens, particular those who are African American and Latino, are decked out in designer fashions and sporting extravagant jewelry. They believe that, with money and the things money buys, they can transform themselves. They want to distance themselves from the types of perceptions and attributions that were made about me that day at the law school. So, they devote themselves to trying to dress like and possess the items that they associate with being rich. Ironically, members of the upper classes enjoy the privilege of not having to worry about others seeing them as upper- or upper-middle-class—they take it for granted. They can even comfortably "dress down" because they don't feel that they have anything to prove. There is no mark of shame from which they are desperately trying to escape.

"When you live on the wrong side of the tracks, it's like being branded with an iron that says you're trash." Having lived her whole life in poverty, Tawny was intimately familiar with the devaluation that came with her class status. "It's hard enough not having things that I want, like enough hot water to take a long, soaking bath whenever I want. Did I tell you about that? I'm only allowed three baths a week and I can't even fill the tub all the way. But even worse than not having things is having the knowledge that people look down on me. I'm worthless in their eyes—I'm dirt. That's what really hurts more than anything else." For Tawny, being poor limited the things she had, but it also limited who she was, or who others perceived her to be. In the literal sense, her restricted baths were a symptom of her economic deprivation. But they also were powerful symbols of the ways in which she felt devalued by the judgments of the world around her. Because she was poor, she was made to feel dirty or less valuable than those of more privileged classes.

Societal devaluation tied to class can have a powerful effect on adolescents who are prone to violence. Coming from a working-class family, Timothy Ryan appeared to struggle intensely with the devaluation related to his class status. Recall his remark about the girl he had raped, "that rich bitch." This reference revealed that for Timothy, class—and more specifically his sense of devaluation related to class—was an organizing variable in his act of violence. The devaluation he experienced in terms of class was one more way in which he felt inferior, and one more factor to bear in mind when trying to develop a clear picture of the anatomy of his violence.

Gay, Lesbian, and Bisexual Youth

The vast majority of gay, lesbian, and bisexual youth suffer profoundly from societal devaluation, and for the most part they suffer in silence. The struggles these youth face are tragically reflected in the fact that, while it is estimated that 10% of the U.S. adolescent population are gay and lesbian, between 30 and 40% of all youth suicides are committed by gay and lesbian youth. This disturbing statistic reveals the depth of the pain many of these adolescents feel, and this pain is directly tied to the societal devaluation that afflicts anyone in this society who is not heterosexual.

Within U.S. society there is a deeply entrenched assumption of heterosexuality. When speaking to little boys and girls, it is common for adults to make seemingly "innocent" comments that assume that all children will someday grow up to date and marry someone of the opposite gender. How many times have we heard someone say, for example, to a little girl, "You'll marry a nice young man one day," or about a little boy, "He's going to make some woman really happy one day." From the time they are very young, little kids are conditioned to believe that the only viable option available for them is one of heterosexual union. For children who are gay, lesbian, or bisexual this assumption can have devastating consequences. Initially, it generates extreme confusion in young children who never receive any acknowledgment that same-sex relationships are even a possibility—let alone that they are a valid, normal possibility. After confusion, these kids develop a deep sense of shame because most conclude early on that the feelings they have must be wrong and unnatural and that therefore there must be something wrong with them. Indeed, most gay, lesbian, and bisexual kids often are exposed to homophobic comments and actions that much more directly express contempt toward anything that is nonheterosexual.

Ellie knew from the time she was 7 that she was drawn to other little girls rather than boys. When she was 8 she was crushed when her best friend said she wanted to marry one of their classmates, who was a little boy. Ellie felt jealous because in her heart she wanted to marry Christie herself when they grew up. But Ellie hid her feelings. At 8, she did not have a vocabulary to explain what she already understood: that it was not okay for her to have romantic feelings toward other little girls.

> "My family is really homophobic. Once we were in a park, and my father saw two men holding hands and he made us move away. He said they were perverts. I felt sick to my stomach when that happened because I knew that what he was saying was that I was a pervert. Even though he didn't know he was talking about me, I knew."

Many gay, lesbian, and bisexual youth internalize feelings of self-hatred in response to the relentless heterosexist and homophobic conditioning they receive that teaches them that who they are is wrong. Is it any wonder that so many of these kids turn violent toward themselves, either poisoning their bodies with drugs or making more overt attempts to end their lives? "I just couldn't live with the shame any longer," Roberto explained.

> "I was living a secret life. I was in love with a guy named Pete, and I hated myself for it. I couldn't stay away from him. I guess he was my first love. But I hated myself for it. I knew my family would never accept me as a gay person. They would rather I was dead than have me be gay. So, I wanted to be dead. It was easier than having to face their disgust, and it was easier than having to live a lie. I still wish I had pulled it off. I have to tell you, I'll probably try again."

For adolescents who are in a state of questioning with regard to sexual orientation, there is no breathing room, no space to take a deep breath and reflect. There is no margin for error. In a society that promotes heterosexuality, simply expressing doubt about one's sexual orientation can be quite painful and costly. Closeted gay, lesbian, bisexual, and questioning youth are often forced to live double lives. They have to wear masks that support the presumption and privilege of heterosexuality while living trapped between the fear of being found out and the anxiety of wanting to be wholly integrated human beings. Unlike girls, or people of color whose physical presence can trigger "politically correct behavior and rhetoric" from adversaries, which can provide a type of shield from insult and assault, many gay, lesbian, and bisexual youth are not so lucky. Many, unfortunately, are relegated to the position of undignified witnesses to others' homophobia, hatred, and threats to do physical harm to anyone who is presumed to be anything but heterosexual. These often experienced but seldom acknowledged experiences leave many gay, lesbian, bisexual, and questioning youth overcome with despair and devaluation. Ironically, any manifestation of their suffering is usually dismissed or attributed to their being "weird, queer, or mixed up." No matter how complex the difficulties with devaluation are for gay, lesbian, bisexual and questioning youth, a firm declaration of their heterosexuality is believed to be the best remedy.

DEVALUATION AND THE EXPRESSION OF VIOLENCE

A fascinating relationship exists between experiences with devaluation and how adolescents ultimately express their violence. Among violent adolescents we have observed interesting differences in how white males, males of color, and females of all races unleash their violence.

In terms of race and gender, white male adolescents are socially privileged. Racist and sexist conditioning socializes almost all white males to believe that the world is theirs for the taking and, as such, they are justified in using tactics of domination and aggression to fulfill their needs and desires. For males of color, racially they are conditioned to see themselves as second-class citizens in a world that expects them to serve, not to rule. Yet, on the basis of their gender, they, like white males, are taught to view themselves as superior to females. From this perspective they are conditioned to use tactics of domination and aggression to fulfill their needs and desires. In particular, they are socialized to view girls as objects who exist to fulfill male desires.

Within a patriarchal culture, females are conditioned to subjugate their own needs and desires and to accept a place of subservience beneath men. Few girls graduate into adulthood without having internalized some of the broader messages that teach them to silence their voices, redirect their gazes, and accept an identity that is defined by "serving others." This socialization is more intense for females of color who get multiple layers of this conditioning on the basis of gender and race.

The influence of the socialization processes on how adolescents express their violence is intriguing. It is significant, for example, that all of the perpetrators in the wave of mass school shootings have been white males. It seems beyond coincidence that no boys of color or girls of any race have channeled their violence in this manner. This is not to suggest that males of color and girls of all races do not become violent. They do. But they channel their violence in very different ways. For the white male shooters of Paducah (KY), Jonesboro (AR), Pearl (MS), Springfield (OR), and Littleton (CO) there was an audacity to their violence that reflects the entitlement that is part of white male socialization. Focusing their attacks on their schools revealed a boldness. These boys weren't just targeting individuals, but an entire institution and, in fact, the whole of society. And yet, if this is true, it begs the question, why would these young boys feel such rage against society as a whole? Especially since, as white males, they held privileged positions within this very society. Or did they?

It is our view that—with these boys—the forces of racist and sexist socialization collided with their personal experiences with situational devaluation. On the one hand, they felt the pain of feeling rejected and shamed by other kids, and in some cases by their families as well. And yet, they also had been raised in a culture that had conditioned them to believe they were better than everyone else—that they were superior. Imagine the contradiction between these two levels of experience. This is a clash we often observe among adult white males who have failed to succeed professionally or economically. These men suffer from profound shame because their personal failure is intensified by the humiliation of knowing that as white males they had the benefit of broad-based social opportunities and privileges that no other groups have. At least for those men of color and women of all races who fail professionally or economically, while this failure is painful (especially for men who are taught to believe their worth is measured by their economic success), it is partially tempered by the knowledge that the deck was stacked against them from the beginning. This provides some buffer against the conclusion that one's failure is solely attributable to personal weakness.

For white males who receive messages suggesting they are superior, and yet whose personal experiences involve feelings of profound rejection and inadequacy, the schism may be enough to generate a sense of shame, which is at the heart of devaluation. Moreover, this devaluation, if it remains unaddressed and unhealed, may lead to a deep sense of rage (in this case a rage against the world for not fulfilling its promise of absolute power and privilege). This globalized rage is especially dangerous because as white males, even if they feel their personal experiences don't measure up to the promises of power and glory, they still operate according to the view the world is theirs for the taking. There is a comfort they have in the world at large, perhaps a sense of believing they are "owed" something by the world. Is it any wonder that when their rage finally erupts into violence, their target is "the world," or the symbolic world as represented through a primary societal institution (like a school)? And is it any wonder that their form of violence is often broad, grandiose, and indiscriminate?

This may also explain why almost all serial killers are white males. These killers select targets who are virtual strangers. Their victims are not personal targets. In one sense, their victim is society at large. While the killer's literal victim is an individual person, it is the whole of society who is victimized by the mass terror these killers breed. The same dynamics occur in cases of homegrown terrorism. Again, the perpetrators have all been white males. Consider one of the most well-publicized cases, the Oklahoma City bombing. Clearly the intended target was society (represented as a federal building), and the killing was mass, generalized, and indiscriminate. This is consistent with the globalized rage that stems from the white male orientation toward the world.

For males of color, like white males, their acts of violence tend to be externalized toward others, but more often than not, these others are their "symbolic selves." The alarming rates of black-on-black homicide, particularly among young urban males, depict the complex intersection between race and gender. Literally speaking, these kids are lashing out and killing others, which is consistent with a masculine orientation. Yet, these "others" are their own brothers—in a sense, themselves. Many of these kids are simultaneously committing both homicide and suicide. We would find it highly unusual for any male youth of color to direct his violence in the way that the white male school shooters have. While kids of color may have even more reason to feel rage against society, at least whatever slights they endure from the world around them are consistent with their social programming, which teaches them to never expect anything better. They may be treated as if they are "less than," which may hurt, but it also is consistent with the dominant story about who they are. Most kids of color grow up never expecting much of anything from the world, which tempers the sense of disillusionment that may arise when the world fails them. Hence, most kids of color would never contemplate an attack upon a whole school because it would defy the very socialization process that teaches them the world was never theirs in the first place.

An argument could be made that, to some extent, males of color do in fact lash out against the world, but it's the world as it has been defined for them through racist conditioning. Within this scheme, that which constitutes "the world" is much more local, immediate, and tightly defined than it is for white males.

Many years ago, we knew a young black male, Barry, who grew up and lived in a fairly insular neighborhood within a much larger city. We will never forget the day that we tried to encourage Barry, who was a talented artist, to accept a job in another city that paid a much higher salary than his present job, with opportunities for advancement. But Barry refused it flatly. He explained that he was going to spend the remainder of his life in his neighborhood of origin. "I suppose everything I need is right here. There's no need to venture out." While we respected Barry's right to make this decision, there was a part of his choice that didn't seem like it had been a choice at all. We could not help but wonder in what ways Barry's complacency, or lack of ambition, was a barometer of his deprivation. Having grown up with so little and having been socialized as a black person to expect so little, perhaps Barry was merely conforming to the social-psychological boundaries that had been established for him within a racist society.

As a function of their racial devaluation, few youth of color identify with society's institutions. They see these institutions as part of the white world, which is not their world. This in part explains why many urban youth of color are ambivalent about performing well academically in school. To do so often invites criticism from peers who label this success as being "too white" and as "selling out to the white power." This type of allegation makes it clear that these kids associate school with the white world, which is not their world. The line that divides them is sharply drawn, which is why we would not expect youth of color to focus their violence against schools (i.e., society at large), for example.

For girls of all colors, their violence is most likely to be internalized—to be directed inwardly against themselves, which is consistent with the socialization they receive that teaches them they have no right to expect anything of the world, and whatever failures and disappointments they suffer, they have only themselves to blame. Hence, girls are much more likely to cut themselves, develop eating disorders and drug/alcohol addictions, and commit suicide.

Hence, rather then reflecting a breaking out of social constraints, to some extent, expressions of adolescent violence are a reformulation of societal pressures that are grounded in the complex intersection of race, class, and gender politics. For those young people who are compelled toward acts of violence, the specific manifestations of this violence are largely mitigated by the socialization they receive in terms of broader dimensions of the sociocultural context.

CONCLUSION

It is important to remember that devaluation is but one aggravating factor that ultimately contributes to adolescent violence. There are millions of teenagers who endure painful experiences with devaluation, both situational and societal, and yet most do not resort to violence. We believe that the issue of what divides "those who do" from "those who don't" lies in the complex interaction of the *four aggravating factors* that constitute our model—of which devaluation is only the first. In the next chapter we discuss the second aggravating factor, the disruption or erosion of community.

CHAPTER 3

• • • • • • •

Disruption of Community

The dark circles under Carmen's eyes reflected her recent ordeal. She had passed out in the elevator of her dormitory, the result of massive consumption of alcohol mixed with prescription drugs. She was rushed to the hospital, where her stomach was pumped. Several days later, she sat in our office looking frail and forlorn.

"I don't think I was trying to kill myself, but I think it would be better if I had died."

Carmen's sense of hopelessness and despair filled the small therapy room. By most measures, her life was full of potential and hope. She possessed intelligence, beauty, charm, and came from a loving and secure family. It was hard to understand why a girl who had so much to live for would feel better off if she were dead.

Carmen's physical beauty was captivating. Even in spite of the trauma she had recently endured, her smooth brown skin, sculpted cheekbones, and chocolate brown eyes were striking. But there was more to Carmen than her radiant physical beauty. She was gentle, authentic, and a bright student with a near perfect academic record. She had a loving family who adored her. Both her parents and her older sister seemed devastated by Carmen's overdose. They had vowed to do whatever they could to support Carmen and help her recover.

Despite the many positive things that Carmen had in her favor, she was plagued by an inner pain that was driving her to self-destruction. We needed to peel back the layers and see the suffering that hid just beyond the pretty picture that the outside world saw. Once we did this, we discovered that Carmen was haunted by a profound disruption to her sense of community.

DEFINING COMMUNITY

Our work with violent adolescents has helped us to appreciate how the disruption of community is a key aggravating factor underpinning adolescent violence. Before describing the impact of the disruption of community on teens, we think it's important to spend some time clarifying what we mean when we use the term "community."

Defining the concept of community is difficult because everyone has an idea of what the term means, yet a clear, concrete definition remains somewhat elusive. Whenever we ask people to share with us their image of what community is, the responses we get are often general and vague. Typical responses include "a group of people united by a common interest," "a group of people who live in a specific area," "a group of people who share a common racial, ethnic, or religious identity and are bonded together on this basis," and "a physical place, like a community center, where people can come together and just hang out." These definitions touch upon important aspects of what community is, and yet they fail to reflect the emotional, psychological, and spiritual dimensions of community. These definitions do not represent the part of community that involves *feelings*—feelings of belonging, rootedness, identity, connection, safety, security, familiarity, caring, and hope.

Through our work with violent adolescents, we have developed a view of community that emphasizes both its physical, tangible dimensions and its emotional, psychological, and spiritual ones. In short, we believe community is a "place" where adolescents feel a sense of belonging and connection with others in a special way. It's a place where they learn about who they are. It's where they begin to develop a sense of identity and a vision of how they "fit" in the world around them. Community is a place where adolescents can find answers to life's many difficult and complicated questions. It is a place where adolescents find comfort when they are overcome with despair, a place where they feel accepted. It is a community that provides adolescents with a sense of safety, security, and meaningful relatedness with others. It is "in community" that teens derive the comfort and familiarity that comes from being surrounded and protected by others who care about them. Community provides a buffer against the trials and tribulations of life. It can foster tremendous resiliency in the face of enormous adversity. It nurtures pro-social development by acting as an incubator for the cultivation of qualities such as compassion, caring, cooperation, collaboration, and conscience. Community is "home."

When teens have a strong sense of community, it serves as a buffer against devaluation. Conversely, where there is an absence or a disruption in community, adolescents are more vulnerable to the trauma of devaluation. In fact, the disruption or erosion of community in the lives of young people can, in and of itself, constitute a form of devaluation.

DISRUPTION OF COMMUNITY

Among adolescents who become violent, the disruption of community is almost always evident. To the extent that community is a synonym for home, violent teens suffer from a chronic state of "psychological homelessness" (Hardy, 1997). Their existence is ravaged by an existential alienation that cuts deep into the core of their being, wounding every dimension of their person. The disruption of community in the lives of adolescents robs them of the security, connectedness, acceptance, and identity that they desperately need. When their sense of community is disrupted, something basic to their humanity is deeply wounded.

With the disruption of community, many of the positive qualities that community nurtures are disrupted as well, such as a sense of compassion and caring for others. It is through community that people learn how to care for others, how to cooperate and collaborate, and how to negotiate the complications that accompany being connected to others in a meaningful way. When teens suffer from a disruption of community, their acquisition of these important relational skills is assaulted. Is it any wonder then that so many adolescents struggle with forming caring attachments? Is it a surprise that some of them seem to lack altogether a sense of conscience? After all, when a person suffers from an absence of community, he or she also suffers from an absence of conscience. The two go hand in hand. In the case of Timothy Ryan, for example, the disruptions in his sense of community created corresponding cracks in his capacity to relate empathetically to others. Because he felt as if he had been abandoned and betrayed within his family, he experienced the world as a rejecting place. He did not perceive others as recognizing or responding in caring ways to his feelings and needs. As a result, he not only became narcissistically consumed with his own needs, but he also did not learn how to recognize and respond with caring or compassion to others' feelings or needs. Had he had a more secure sense of community growing up, he would have felt the comfort of his parents nurturing him. Because that was not his reality, his capacity for empathy was not cultivated, leading to the type of absence of conscience that enabled him to look into the eyes of his victims and beat them mercilessly. It was the absence of conscience that made it possible for him to feel the breath of the girl on his face, and feel her heartbeat pressed against his body, to hear her cries echoing in his ear while he raped her remorselessly. It was the absence of conscience that made all of this possible. To be alienated from community is to be alienated from one's humanity, and when this occurs, the potential for violence increases dramatically.

Adolescents who suffer from disruptions of their sense of community also experience the most deadly consequence of all—a loss of hope. It is through community that a sense of hope is created. Community provides adolescents with a sense of their past as well as a vision for their future. James Garbarino (1999) talks about the "lack of a future orientation," which is common among violent teens. We believe that chronic massive disruptions in one's sense of community assault one's capacity to have a future orientation. Those who don't feel connected to others lack a sense of rootedness and, hence, a feeling of relatedness to their historical ties. Without this, they also lack a meaningful identification with a future. A future orientation requires a connection to one's past, which feeds a vision for one's future. Our roots—both the bitter and the sweet ones—give birth to our dreams, and ultimately ignite a sense of purpose. They inspire us to have something for which to strive, hope, and aspire. All of these "essentials to our being" are provided and nurtured in community. Adolescents who have suffered profound disruptions to their sense of community suffer from a deprivation of hope and vision regarding their future.

LEVELS OF COMMUNITY

There are three levels of community that adolescents participate in that are vital to their growth and development. We have noted, among adolescents who become violent, that they suffer from the disruption of community on at least two, and usually all three, levels. It seems to be this cumulative impact of disruption at more than one level that puts teens most at risk for violence.

At the first level are *primary communities,* which refer to families, however one defines family. We realize that calling a family a community defies popular notions of the term "community." Few people think of families when they use the term community, and yet all of the properties that are typically associated with community apply to families. For example, families are groups of people who are united in a special way and who share a common interest. It is in families that individuals experience their first sense of belonging to something that is greater than themselves. It is in families where people get their first sense of rootedness and connection. This is where one's initial identity is established. Families—at least when they are healthy—are places that individuals can turn to find comfort, acceptance, and a feeling of "home." So, while it may be unconventional, we believe that families are the first community, the "primary community."

Just beyond the level of primary communities are *extended communities,* which include neighborhoods, schools, churches, synagogues, temples, civic groups, community centers, and so forth. Extended communities most closely approximate conventional views of what community represents. Hence, it is fairly easy to relate to this level of community. Within extended communities people experience a sense of themselves as connected to a clearly defined group that exists beyond their families. Such groups exist at the local level, in the sense that the borders of the community are clearly identifiable. The other distinguishing characteristic of extended communities is that they are usually connected to physical locations (e.g., schools, houses of worship, community centers).

The third level consists of *cultural communities.* This refers to the communities that adolescents have membership in on the basis of their race, ethnicity, gender, social class, sexual orientation, mental/physical ability, and religion. Like extended communities, cultural communities also extend an individual's identity beyond his or her family. However, unlike the situation with extended communities, cultural communities have *intangible* borders. It is within the cultural community that boys and girls, for example, learn what it means, at least according to society, to be a "boy" or "girl." Obviously, some of this socialization occurs within primary and extended communities, but it has been our experience that the larger portion of this get refined within the cultural community. We don't wish to imply here that the dynamics of the cultural community are limited to gender socialization. The scope and impact of the cultural community are broad. It is through this level of community, for example, that we, as human beings, get acutely acquainted with ourselves through the prisms of class, race, ethnicity, and so forth.

FORCES THAT DISRUPT COMMUNITY

There are many different forces that can disrupt community at all levels. Some of these influences are discussed below for each level of community.

Disruption of Primary Communities

The basic building block of a sense of community at the primary level consists of parent–child relationships. There are several ways in which parent–child relationships are disrupted.

Abuse

Parental abuse of children and adolescents profoundly disrupts the parent–child bond. One of the serious dangers of abuse is that it teaches young people directly that violence is acceptable. Abusive parents convey the message that it is okay to use force, domination, and aggression to solve problems, to control others, and to express feelings like anger and frustration. While not all abused children and adolescents are doomed to become abusers themselves, or to utilize tactics of aggression to handle everyday living, the risk of these tendencies is higher among those who are victims of violence and aggression.

In some perverse way, many children and adolescents "prefer" abuse to neglect because at least, with abuse, there is a form of acknowledgment that they exist. This was personified for us by a boy who told us, "I know he hits me [referring to his father], but he don't really mean any harm . . . It's just who he is, and I know he hits me 'cause he cares." While the abuse was obviously painful and destructive, at least it was a form of acknowledgment to this boy that his father noticed him. With neglect, no such acknowledgment exists. Such parents wound their children by denying them altogether.

Of course, the "acknowledgment" that comes with abuse is dysfunctional. It's more akin to how a person might recognize a chair rather than recognizing another human being. It's possible to see and recognize a chair, to even devote some energy toward interacting with it (i.e., sitting in it), but there is nothing inherent in the interaction that acknowledges that the chair has feelings, rights, or needs. The chair is simply an object, a thing that is there to serve. So, while abusive parents provide some cursory acknowledgment of their children's existence, the acknowledgment occurs through aggression and trauma, which translates into a deeper level of emotional and psychological neglect and abandonment.

Neglect

Neglect consists of ignoring children and adolescents and, therefore, failing to provide them with essential physical, emotional, and/or psychological sustenance. This can occur overtly, as with parents who physically abandon and thus neglect their kids in every way possible. It also can occur covertly, as in the case of parents who remain physically present but still neglect their children's emotional, psychological, and physical needs to varying degrees. When parents neglect their kids, they are in effect denying their children's very existence. As one severely neglected 12-year-old client told us during a therapy session, "My mom doesn't notice me at all. I could be dead and she wouldn't notice." When kids experience this level of rejection, not only do they suffer from a disruption of their primary-level community, but they also suffer from devaluation. Another example of neglect was depicted in the movie *Harold and Maude*. The film portrays a young boy who is virtually ignored by his mother. In his desperation to get his mother to notice him, he goes to absurd lengths, including an attempt to hang himself in her presence. Because his mother is incapable of acknowledging her son's existence, even this extreme act fails to capture her attention. Even in the face of his obvious attempt at asphyxiation, she speaks to him about something irrelevant and superficial. Clearly, his mother does not actually see him. The casual, nonaffected comment she utters is grossly inappropriate in light of Harold's behavior. The message within the message is "You, Harold, are totally invisible to me. I don't see you at all. You don't exist in my world." Harold is a classic child of neglect, and it requires little effort to see the ways in which this neglect is highly devaluing.

The topic of neglect is complicated because the neglect can be manifested in different ways and to varying degrees. The reality is that a large majority of parents have direct contact with their children, either in terms of living in the same household or speaking with and having their children visit with them on a regular basis. Most parents have a physical presence in their kids' lives. Similarly, most parents also attend to their child's basic physical needs. Yet, there are more subtle forms of neglect that can have damaging consequences for young people, such as emotional neglect. Fathers in particular are prone to being emotionally neglectful. For example, parents who work extended hours may provide for their kids, but by virtue of their demanding work schedules, fail to be emotionally available. This may have been a dynamic that affected both Eric Harris and Dylan Klebold. While both boys lived within "intact" two-parent family households where their parents were attentive to their physical needs, they may have been emotionally neglected. The fact that there seemed to be little parental awareness of the warning signs (e.g., extended isolated hours spent in their basements constructing bombs, the rage and alienation they experienced at school) that both boys emitted prior to their killing spree suggests a lack of meaningful connection between them and their parents.

It also is common for loving, devoted parents to inadvertently hurt their kids by failing to recognize and encourage their strengths, by failing to display affection, or by making comments or statements that, while intended to be corrective and helpful, have the consequence of disturbing or disrupting their fragile sense of self-esteem. For example, we recently had a parent in therapy who told her 13-year-old daughter, "I'd better not find you snacking on those cookies. Your weight is getting totally out of control." While the comment was motivated by concern for the daughter, it had a devastating impact on the girl's already low sense of self-regard.

Despite the fact that we live in a increasingly diverse society, most people still think of a "normal family" as "the 1950s image of a white, affluent, nuclear family headed by a breadwinner/father and supported by a full-time homemaker/mother" (Walsh, 1998, p. 15). Therefore, when we see families that match this image, we tend to assume that these families are "normal" and "healthy." We give these families the benefit of the doubt. Rarely if ever do we look beneath the surface to see what's really happening on the inside of the family. For the most part, we are deceived by the structure of the family, and fail to consider the emotional quality of the family relationships. As a result, it is sometimes hard to recognize how these families might be failing to provide children and adolescents with a strong, stable primary community. This became clear for us when we were presenting a workshop on violent adolescents to a group of therapists. In the middle of our presentation we were interrupted by a woman from the audience who was visibly irritated with our ideas. She said to us:

"I'm having a hard time with what you're saying. I don't think that all kids who become problem kids are suffering from a disruption of community. I work in a school, and I'm thinking of the family of a boy in our school. He's a troubled boy, to say the least, but there isn't really any good reason for it. He has community all around him. Our school is one of the best in the county. And he comes from a good family. He's got his mother and father and his grandparents living with him. He is surrounded by people who are committed to raising him well. But in spite of all that he acts up all the time. I think it's just who he is. Sometimes, kids are just trouble. That's it."

As we continued to seek more information from this woman, she eventually disclosed that she thought this little boy probably had a hearing disability, but she could not find out for sure because his parents would not authorize hearing tests. She explained that the father was a "fire-and-brimstone" preacher who did not believe in interfering with God's plan. If his son had difficulty in hearing, so be it. The boy's mother had been treated for depression, which was so severe that on one occasion she had to be hospitalized when this boy was only 4 years old. We cite this example because it illustrates nicely how our biases about what a "good" family looks like can sometimes make it hard to see when a family is failing to provide a stable community for a child. As was the case with this little boy, while his parents were physically present, they seemed to be completely absent emotionally, which no doubt disrupted his sense of primary community.

Sometimes the disruption of primary community can be subtle and hard to detect outright. There is ample evidence to suggest, for example, that Theodore Kaczynski (the Unabomber) was a man who suffered from severe disruption of community beginning at infancy; however, some of the disruptions were not readily obvious at first glance. To begin with, after only a few weeks of life, little Ted became ill and was hospitalized for several months. In accordance with standard hospital protocol during the 1950s, he was placed in an isolation unit, where he was deprived of all contact with his family. This severely undermined the development of a stable sense of community at the primary level. In fact, the only human contact Ted had during his months of hospitalization was via the sterile and perfunctory tasks that were administered by nurses who changed his diapers, fed him, and performed various medical procedures. The months during his illness and hospitalization disrupted Ted's primary community during a critical period of his development. Extensive bonding and attachment studies have since demonstrated how vital it is to have consistent physical and emotional nurturance from a primary caretaker during the early stages of life. These early experiences provide the template upon which all future connections and relationships are based. Infants who are deprived of consistent, loving contact with a primary caretaker fail to develop the secure attachments that are a prerequisite for healthy relationship formation and development in later life.

In Ted's case, it seemed that the early disruption of his primary community had taken its toll. His mother reported that the child she had known prior to the illness was vastly different from the child who returned home after many months in the hospital. A once happy and smiley baby had become distant, introverted, and withdrawn. There was a newfound distance and disconnection between mother and son that had not existed prior to Ted's illness and subsequent hospitalization. Moreover, the strains that now existed between Ted and his family never really improved with time. It seemed that Ted had suffered tragic effects of the disruption of his primary community in infancy, which may have disrupted bonding and attachment during a critical period of development, thereby contributing to future patterns of isolation and disconnection.

Throughout childhood, Ted's intellect was indisputable, as was his lack of social engagement. Having few friends, he spent most of his time alone reading scientific magazines, studying math, and exploring the outdoors. When there is an absence of community early in life, one is deprived of critical opportunities to acquire and refine basic life skills, which then becomes a detriment to the establishment and maintenance of community later in life. In Ted's case, as an undergraduate at Harvard his patterns toward social isolation persisted. Stemming from the absence of community during his earlier years, he had failed to develop basic life skills, including how to connect and relate to others socially. Hence, he had few, if any, friends and was regarded by his peers as a loner. Despite his obvious intellectual brilliance he remained socially awkward and disconnected throughout his life, which was exemplified by his frequent retreats to his wilderness cabin in Montana. Ted lived a quiet, rugged, back-to-the-basics existence for months at a time, completely isolated from other human beings.

Although Ted Kaczynski's 18-year-long spree of violence did not begin during his adolescence, his life provides an excellent illustration of the relationship that often exists between the disruption of community (for even its absence) and violence. Ted's capacity to commit cold, calculated acts of violence against his fellow human beings was inevitably facilitated by his general alienation from and lack of meaningful connections with others. In light of the socioemotional vacuum that Ted lived in, it requires minimal effort to see how he was able to hurt other living beings with so little regard for the suffering he caused.

Separation/Divorce

Parental separation and divorce are other common ways in which children experience the disruption of their primary community. Depending upon how parents handle their separation or divorce, the experience can contribute greatly to the children's feeling neglected, abandoned, and/or abused. The fact that 75% of children rarely see the noncustodial parent after their parents' divorce equates to neglect and abandonment in the minds of many children. Moreover, when couples undergo bitter, vicious divorces, children often are caught in the crossfire between warring parties, which is abusive. Their unfortunate position in the middle of their parents' hostility means that children hear one or both parents say ugly things about the other. Some parents also use their children as pawns and bargaining chips in their battles. When this occurs, it is devastating to children because it reduces them to objects and neglects their needs.

Death

Finally, the death of a parent is another way in which community at the primary level can be disrupted. Following the death of a parent, children and adolescents often feel abandoned. Except in the case of suicide, parents who die do not intentionally leave their children. But for those kids who no longer have their parents around to nurture and guide them, they often feel as if they have been abandoned.

It was during our third session with Carmen that we learned the story of her childhood and how she had lost both of her birth parents in a brutal attack. Carmen was born to José and Maya Santiago, a young couple who lived in a small village in Peru. When Carmen was 6 years old, her parents were killed by guerrillas of the Shining Path. "I don't remember my parents dying. I just remember being in an orphanage and crying for my mother. I remember feeling so lonely." The death of Carmen's parents disrupted her primary community beyond repair. While her parents were not responsible for their death, to 6-year-old Carmen, their loss was experienced as abandonment. According to Carmen, the next year that she spent living in an orphanage "was the loneliest, most empty year of my life. I felt abandoned in a cold, ugly world without anyone to love and comfort me."

Disruption of Extended Communities

Extended communities can be disrupted by external factors, such as harsh economic conditions, or by internal factors that undermine the solidarity and direction of a group. Many urban schools, for example, are disrupted by a lack of access to economic resources, which undermines their capacity to create nurturing, healthy, progressive environments for students (Kozol, 1991). In other cases, an organization like a church or community center might experience a disruption of community rooted in destructive internal politics that leads to struggles for power and sabotages a strong sense of cohesiveness, positive spirit, and community among the congregation or staff.

When the guerrillas of the Shining Path attacked the village that Carmen had been born and raised in, not only was her primary community brutally destroyed, but also her extended one as well. When she was placed within the orphanage that was miles from her village, she mourned for her parents and for the many people who had loved and cared for her. She was robbed of the hugs she used to look forward to from the women who sat with her mother. She was robbed of the laughter she enjoyed during the large communal celebrations. She was robbed of a sense of connection to a collective who was not her family but whom she loved and relied upon nonetheless.

Natural disasters, such as earthquakes, floods, hurricanes, and tornadoes, are another way in which extended communities can be disrupted. When hurricane Andrew hit south Florida in 1991, it wiped out entire neighborhoods. Nature's wrath did not distinguish between the mansions inhabited by the wealthy and the trailers that were home to the poor. The force of nature leveled extended communities, irrespective of socioeconomic standing, and left everyone with the painful task of having to rebuild from the rumble.

Outcast Status as Disruption of Community at the Extended Level

The previous examples have all considered how entire extended communities can be disrupted, which clearly has a damaging effect upon adolescents who have membership in these communities. It also is possible for a teen to experience a much more personal sense of disruption of community at the extended level. Before Eric Harris and Dylan Klebold waged their brutal attack, Columbine High School was an intact extended community. This was a school that provided its students with all the benefits of economic prosperity. This was a school that was characterized by "school spirit" and where most of the kids received a solid, well-rounded education. In all likelihood, most of the students attending Columbine felt a positive connection to their school. Yet, this was not the case for Eric and Dylan. For these two boys, their sense of extended community at school was disrupted by the intense and persist isolation, ostracism, and rejection they felt from their peers. Routinely called names and taunted by other students who perceived them as uncool and weird, Eric and Dylan were the types of kids who often fall between the cracks in school like Columbine. Where everything looks good on the surface, and where most students do well, kids like Eric and Dylan are often ignored as social misfits who don't fit in but who are assumed to pose no real harm. And yet, as history now indicates, the pain they felt in response to their lack of community at the extended level was unbelievably intense and acutely dangerous.

Bullying as Disruption of Community at the Extended Level

Bullying, particularly in schools, has reached epidemic proportions (Garbarino & Delara, 2003; Garrett, 2003; Wessler & Preble, 2003). It has become such a chronic problem in schools that many administrators and school boards are developing stringent zero-tolerance policies to address the problem. In schools where bullying is prevalent, it is difficult for students to feel a sense of safety and security. School, unfortunately, becomes a terror zone. When bullying is present, it has a major deleterious affect on children's extended community. Like youth violence, bullying feeds off of itself. In more instances than not, a child who has been bullied will eventually become a bully. In a school culture and climate where bullying exists, providing students with a healthy extended community with all of its benefits becomes virtually impossible.

FORCES THAT DISRUPT CULTURAL COMMUNITIES

Cultural communities are disrupted by the forces of racism, homophobia, sexism, classism, anti-Semitism, and so forth. After living in the orphanage for almost a year, Carmen was eventually adopted by a wealthy couple, the Brodys, from New York. In one way, the adoption was a new beginning for her. It was a chance to restore her disrupted sense of primary and extended community. But on another level, one that was invisible to her parents and most of people she interacted with, this was the beginning of a persistent, intensely painful assault upon her sense of cultural community.

Carmen's new family loved her from the moment they saw her. Their hearts could not have opened any wider had she been born to them. And yet, the reality was that she and her new family inhabited two extremely different worlds. They were a white, wealthy North American family. Carmen was a poor South American Indian from a developing country. She had lived all of her life until that point in a small rural mountain village. When she first met her new parents, she did not speak any English.

The Brodys desperately wanted Carmen to forget her past because they assumed it would be too painful for her to remember. Because they believed that focusing on her past would be traumatic, they referred to it sparingly and only in perfunctory ways. Moreover, the Brodys wanted so desperately to make Carmen a genuine member of their family that they did what many white parents do when they adopt children of color: they treated her as if she were white. Instead of acknowledging the differences between them, they sought to minimize these. The family colluded to perpetrate the myth that Carmen was just like them. They taught her English, they taught her Judaism as her new religion, and they never spoke of their racial or class differences. She simply became "one of them."

The desire to incorporate Carmen into their family was admirable, but it was not without problems. It forced Carmen to deny who she was. It forced her to pretend to be someone she was not, which she perceived as a negative message about her identity. As she once stated to us, "It made me feel like it was bad to be me—like I had to be just like them to be okay." It also made it difficult for Carmen to approach her family to discuss the ways in which she was subjected to racial taunts in school that left her feeling devalued. Because the unstated rule in her family was to not talk about their differences, Carmen never felt the comfort to tell her parents how she was often ridiculed by other kids because of her race and her accent.

It's not only kids who have membership in socially devalued groups who experience disruption of community at the cultural level. Sometimes kids who have membership in socially privileged groups also experience a disruption at the cultural level. This occurs when a cultural community manufactures and directs hate toward other groups. For example, when white kids feel racial hatred toward people of color, it prevents them from feeling a genuine positive sense of community in terms of their own racial identity. Whenever identification with a community is based on hatred and intolerance, it creates a false sense of community. A genuine sense of community cannot take root when it built upon the toxic soil that feeds a need to destroy others. Consider an extreme example, the case of Nazi Germany. Germans' nationalistic zeal during the 1930s suggested that they had a strong, cohesive sense of cultural community. And yet this community was rooted in a deep hatred toward Jews. Ultimately one cannot hate others without hating one's own self. As Alice Walker (1989) stated, "You cannot curse a part without damning the whole" (p. 197). Hence, cultural communities that have hate as their central focal point do not truly provide the type of life-sustaining energy that is the essence of community.

In the case of the Columbine High School shooters, Harris and Klebold, their disdain for their classmates was also peppered with racial hatred. Isaiah Schoels was an African American classmate who was apparently targeted because he was black. Before murdering him, Harris and Klebold reportedly taunted him with cruel racial epithets. The fact that they had a relationship with their whiteness based on white supremacy suggested that they did not truly feel a meaningful and secure tie to their whiteness. Hence, in addition to the disruption of community that the two boys experienced at the primary and extended levels, we wonder if they also felt this at the cultural level in terms of race. Those who formulate a sense of community that is based upon hating others are joining together reactively. Those who attempt to achieve a sense of community by directing hate at someone else are disconnected from the very qualities that are essential to the formation and maintenance of genuine community. Their purported unity is a reaction to a deep sense of insecurity about the strength and quality of that unity. The type of community that arises from hatred represents a fundamental denial of all the critical components of community, such as compassion, caring, collaboration, cooperation, and particularly conscience.

CONCLUSION

Devaluation can be a force that assaults community. Moreover, when adolescents suffer from a disruption of community, this can become a source of devaluation. And yet, our picture is still undeveloped. In the next chapter we present and discuss the third aggravating factor associated with adolescent violence, the dehumanization of loss.

CHAPTER 4

• • • • • • •

The Dehumanization of Loss

"It was like everything was happening in slow motion. The man with the gun told my daddy to give him his money. My daddy told him to be cool. He said he didn't have any money 'cause we'd just spent it all in the store. I was holding the bag from the store, and I wanted to lift it up to show the man that my daddy was telling the truth, but I didn't move. The man's eyes were bulging, and veins were popping out around his face. He said, 'Bullshit, man, give me your money . . . I ain't got no time for no fuckin' games.' Daddy said he was gonna go in his pocket and show the man his wallet. He moved slow and pulled out his wallet and opened it. There was a dollar inside. The man freaked out. I don't remember exactly how it happened, but the next thing I remember is seeing my daddy falling. He fell on his knees, and he was holding his chest. Blood was all over his hands. Then he fell forward. I just stood there while the blood went everywhere. It was like I couldn't move. His eyes were open, but he couldn't see me. I knew he was gone."

The expression on Daquon Jackson's face was cold and empty. He recounted the horrific murder of his father without the slightest hint of emotion. Had we not understood the words he were saying, we could easily have assumed he was talking about the weather forecast.

Daquon had never known his mother. She died while giving birth to him. He was 5 years old when he witnessed his father's murder.

After his father died, he lived with his grandparents, who became his legal guardians. According to his grandparents, things were rocky with Daquon from the beginning. During his elementary school years Daquon was quiet and caused little trouble. However, his grades were consistently low, and his teachers were convinced he had a learning disability. By age 8 he was placed in a special education class, where he did not fare much better. When he was 11, he became friends with a boy who was 2 years older and ran with a rough crowd. By the time he was 12 he had been suspended from school five times for fighting. Now, at the age of 14, Mrs. Jackson fearfully explained that she had found a gun in a drawer in Daquon's bedroom.

"I'm just scared to death that he's gonna end up either killin' someone else or getting killed himself. I've already lost a son—I don't want to lose a grandson too. I couldn't take it," Mrs. Jackson said woefully. "I just can't tell you what it did to me to lose my only son. It almost broke me, but I knew I had to stay strong for Daquon. He was so little when his daddy died and he loved him so much. I just prayed to the good Lord to give me the strength to carry on for my grandbaby." Tears welled up in Mrs. Jackson's eyes as she spoke.

"That boy idolized his daddy," stated Mrs. Jackson. "I can't imagine what that child must have gone through after his daddy died, and especially with him seeing how it happened. But he always held it inside. He cried once after the funeral, but I never saw him cry again after that. He was a lot like his daddy, always holding things inside."

When we explored what measures had been taken to help Daquon deal with the brutal murder of his father, Daquon's grandmother said:

"Me and my husband both tried talking to him, but he never let us in. He never said much. Of course, I tried to help him find comfort through the Lord. I always explain to him that when you open your heart to the Lord you find strength and comfort you never dreamed possible. I make sure Daquon goes to church every Sunday, but it's not enough just to go—you have to open yourself to the power of the Lord. I never could get Daquon to understand that. Reverend Robbins has also tried talking to him, tried to help him see the way. I know he likes the Reverend because he's a good man, but he still does not accept Jesus into his life. Finally I got so desperate seeing how he was turning more and more into himself that I took him to a counselor. That didn't do much good either. He refused to say a word. The counselor said he needed time before he could open up. Thing is, it's been 9 years and he still hasn't opened up."

Not only had Daquon suffered terrible losses, but it also seemed that he had lacked the types of experiences that would have allowed him to mourn and heal the pain of his losses. We have found that loss—and more specifically, unacknowledged, unmourned, unhealed loss—is another significant factor underpinning violence among adolescents.

The loss of his father constituted a major disruption in Daquon's primary community. The trauma of this loss was compounded by the fact that Daquon suffered from feelings of devaluation related to the fact that he no longer had either of his parents in his life. Each day in school he was confronted with peers who had the benefit of relationships with at least one, if not both, of their parents. According to his grandmother, when he was in second grade, he lied to several classmates in school about both his parents. For the entire year, according to Mrs. Jackson, Daquon insisted with his classmates that he lived with his mother and father. He lied not only to his peers but to school officials as well. He even fabricated elaborate stories about fun-filled summer vacations as well as holiday and birthday celebrations with his parents.

Mrs. Jackson stated: "This really worried me because his lies became more and more developed. It was as if he believed his own lies. I only found out because the teacher called me. She knew the truth, and she said she was worried this lie might be a sign that he hadn't accepted his parents' death."

"That's not what was happening," Daquon interrupted. "I knew what I was saying wasn't true. I just said it to shut those stupid kids up. They were always going on about 'my daddy is this' or 'my daddy and mama do that.' I was sick of hearing them go on and on about how great their parents were, so I just told them a story that would shut them up. And it worked until that teacher messed it all up."

After we worked intensively with Daquon in therapy, he eventually confirmed our suspicion that devaluation was closely tied to the lies that he told his classmates about his parents. According to Daquon, he was tired of hearing his classmates make references to their parents. From his point of view, his classmates were bragging about their parents, while he had to sit with the pain that both of his parents were dead. To make matters worse, he had never even known his mother. He felt frustrated, jealous, and ashamed. A part of Daquon felt as if he were "less than" them because they had parents who were alive and well, but his parents were dead and gone forever. Although we were concerned about Daquon's lying, we realized that his behavior was his attempt to counteract the sense of devaluation he had suffered with the tragic losses in his primary community.

DIFFERENT TYPES OF LOSS

Our work with loss has led us to make a distinction between tangible and intangible losses. Intangible loss occurs primarily in the emotional and psychological domain. It often entails the loss of respect, dignity, hope, and "voice," just to cite a few examples.

Tangible loss has a physical as well as an emotional-psychological component. We have identified 10 types of tangible loss that commonly afflict adolescents. It is critical to bear in mind that while each of these is characterized by the loss of something physical, there is a corresponding emotional-psychological loss as well that is intangible.

Loss of a Hero

Heroes are the people that we look up to and revere, and with whom we identify. They represent a larger-than-life, idealized image of some aspect of humanity. For example, to many young people, Michael Jordan is a hero. He represents the pinnacle of human athleticism and sportsmanship. As a hero, he is able to capture the imagination of young people around the world and inspire them. He is a role model who provides young people with the vision, hope, and determination to strive to be the best that they can.

The loss of a hero occurs when something happens to undermine that person's idealized status. In other words, the hero "falls from grace." There can be any number of factors that result in "the fall." An athletic hero may become sick or injured, thereby shattering the illusion of superhuman strength and endurance. A moral hero may commit a crime, thereby shattering the illusion of divine virtue and integrity. Whether due to a tragic flaw in their personality or a cruel and unfortunate circumstance, fallen heroes are individuals who have been stripped of their larger-than-life, idealized image. For whatever reason, they go from being semidivine to simply human, and with this demotion comes the loss of the magic, mysticism, and hope that they once created in the minds of those who idolized them. In one sense, they experience some form of devaluation, and by extension those who worshipped and identified with them also incur this devaluation.

Because of the power that heroes have to inspire and motivate, the loss of a hero can be a devastating blow, especially to young people. With the tangible loss of a hero comes the intangible loss of hope, vision, and motivation. When a hero is lost in the eyes of a young person, there is an accompanying sense of disillusionment and emptiness. A little piece of innocence and magic is lost from the world, and in its place the seeds of cynicism and doubt take root.

We were again reminded of the significance of lost heroes in the lives of young people during our work at Markam Middle School. We were originally invited into the school to set up the anti-bullying Bullies to Buddies Program (Hardy, 1999) to help curtail violence, aggression, and bullying among the student body. Three weeks into our work, one of the most popular (and one of the few African American) teachers, Mrs. Chambers, died unexpectedly over a weekend. When school resumed on the ensuing Monday, the unsuspecting students were informed of her untimely death. They were devastated. The emotions of the students and some of the teachers were overwhelming. There were deep guttural sobs and screams from virtually every corner of the building.

We, along with several other colleagues, were asked to provide grief-based emotional-psychological support to the students and teachers. We too were overwhelmed. None of us had ever experienced anything quite so emotionally raw and riveting, especially in a professional setting. Perhaps it was something about seeing the children's innocence and vulnerability unmasked by the harshness of an unanticipated death that sneaked up on us. We quickly found ourselves fighting back tears and working feverishly to maintain some perspective in the midst of all the painful, dreadful, hard-to-hear stories we were hearing about so many of these students' experiences with losses. Not to our surprise, many of these stories were told for the very first time. We were struck not only by the heaviness of the stories but by how they were told, as well. Most of the students reminded us of Daquon in demeanor. They told of the most horrific experiences in such an emotionally detached, stoic, hypnotic-like fashion. Yet, on the other hand, they were clearly and visibly traumatized by Mrs. Chambers's death.

With every child with whom we met, without regard to age, gender, or grade, it became obvious to us that Mrs. Chambers was more than their teacher. For some, she was a second chance for the loving mother they never had, the father who hung in there when things got tough, or the unconditionally loving grandma or pop-pop that they had never known. She was their hero. For many of the African American students, Mrs. Chambers's larger-than-life status represented even more. She was a symbol of hope and inspiration—a reminder to each of them that they should set their goals high and, as she often stated, "keep their heads high because they are not only descendants of slaves but of kings and queens, as well." Her undeniable physical presence as well as the proud and baritone voice in which she spoke was—especially for the black students—an indictment of devaluation. Perhaps Willie, the 13-year-old reputed school terror, provided the best summary of what it means to lose a hero as he angrily but tearfully stated:

"Why did she have to go and die . . . She was the only one who cared about us . . . Who is going to care about us now? . . . I wanted to be a teacher like Mrs. Chambers . . . She always told me that I would make a good teacher . . . [sobbing] I don't wanna be no teacher anymore . . . [lowering his head and crying uncontrollably] I don't wanna be no teacher no more now."

Loss of a Romantic Relationship

Spurred on by raging hormones and unrelenting peer pressure, adolescents are no strangers to experimentation with love and sex. In fact, one of the defining characteristics of adolescence is an emerging "love life." Unfortunately, while burgeoning love relationships are common in adolescence, so also is the phenomenon of "love gone wrong." The scores of chart-topping songs about love torn asunder and love unrequited all seem to reflect the significance of this theme among teenaged listeners. Anyone who listens to the weeping lyrics and woeful melodies that characterize a great deal of teen music is left with little doubt that the loss of a love relationship is one of the most common and painful experiences associated with adolescence. It seems that few teens graduate from their adolescence without having felt the pangs of a broken heart.

A lost love relationship involves more than the obvious tangible loss (in terms of not having that special person there by your side to hug and to hold). It also involves an accompanying intangible loss in terms of hope, dignity, and respect. For example, to most adults, adolescent love relationships represent little more than "puppy love"—an immature, superficial attraction that cannot compare with the intensity, depth, and substance of adult love. When adults minimize the significance of adolescent love relationships (and the pain that arises when they don't work), this exacerbates the intangible aspect of the loss. Not only must adolescents deal with the agony of a love that has been lost or that will never be, but they also must deal with the loss of dignity and respect that comes with having their suffering trivialized by some adults.

Shattered adolescent love relationships are common among youth who are involved in school-related violence. Not only do these experiences constitute disruption of community, and devaluation, but the implications for loss, anger, and rage are profound. We believe that it makes good common sense for those of us working with adolescents to take these relationships very seriously and keep in mind that they may be the first meaningful nonfamilial love relationships that the adolescent has experienced.

Separation and/or Divorce

When a couple is no longer able to maintain a viable relationship and seeks a separation or divorce, it triggers deep-rooted fears within their children regarding their overall sense of security and worth. It is commonplace for young people to worry about any number of issues when their parents separate and/or divorce. Some of these include:

- "What will happen to me?"
- "Will I ever see the parent who is moving out?"
- "Is it my fault?"
- "Don't my parents love me?"
- "Does this mean my family isn't normal anymore?"

While there are healthy ways that parents can handle a separation or divorce so as to minimize the disruption in their children's lives, it is impossible to eliminate the pain associated with losing the family they once knew and the family that will never be again. Irrespective of how unhappy a family situation may have been, and despite whatever steps parents might take to create a smooth transition, the fact remains that a separation or divorce results in the tangible loss of a family as it once existed. Even in the case of a couple that reconciles after a separation, the family is forever changed by the stress and strain that the separation created. It is inevitable that most children will need to mourn for the family they once knew. Furthermore, in addition to the physical loss of the family they once knew, many children experience intangible loss as well. For instance, some children fear they may never be part of a whole happy family, and therefore they suffer from a loss of hope and security. In cases where a separation or divorce is especially bitter and tense, children caught in the crossfire may suffer from a loss of dignity and respect.

Abandonment or Death

In addition to separation and/or divorce, young people can suffer loss in the form of parents (and/or other significant adult figures) who physically abandon them. Abandonment is a deeply wounding event in the lives of young people, because it not only results in the physical loss of a loved one but also breeds a host of complex dynamics that reflect highly painful emotional-psychological losses as well.

When adults abandon children, the result is the immediate and obvious loss of people who were an integral part of those children's lives. This tangible loss creates a void in the relational world of the young people who are left behind. In addition to coping with the tangible loss associated with abandonment, children who are left behind also are confronted with myriad intangible losses as well. For instance, it is common in cases of abandonment for adults who leave to do so abruptly without notification or explanation. The absence of a clear explanation for the departure leaves children to formulate their own reasons. Many assume it was some fault of theirs, some dimension of their character that was flawed, some way in which they simply were unworthy of love. Children who blame themselves in this way suffer from intense feelings of shame and humiliation that are associated with a loss of dignity and respect. They believe that it was some unforgivable shortcoming within them that triggered the abandonment. As a result, abandonment and devaluation are highly interrelated.

Death is similar to the phenomenon of abandonment. In both cases, the loss of a loved one tends to be unexpected, without warning or preparation. In both cases the loved one is completely gone from one's range of vision or contact. The difference is that in the case of death, unlike abandonment, those who are left behind are less likely to blame themselves. While survivors of the deceased sometimes assume their loved one "was taken" as punishment for some failing of theirs, death—more than abandonment—lends itself to the interpretation that bad things just happen and no one is to blame.

Another difference is that in the case of death there is a tendency to idealize the person who died, as in Daquon's case. There is a level of fantasy that can help the person manage the pain of the loss. With abandonment there is a tendency to demonize the person. Moreover, one often struggles with a sense of ambivalence around connection and rage related to the perceived rejection.

Perhaps the most salient difference between death and abandonment is that when a loved one dies, versus choosing to leave, all hope of ever seeing that person again (at least on earth) also dies. In cases of abandonment, some sliver of hope always remains that one day the person who left may either choose to return or could be found. With death, there is the overt tangible loss of the loved one. However, because of the finality of death, there also is a corresponding intangible loss of hope. When someone dies, there is no chance—not even remotely—of being reunited (on earth) with the loved one.

Neglect

In the case of neglect, a parent or other primary caretaker is physically present but fails to provide for his or her child emotionally and functionally (i.e., preparing adequate meals, providing appropriate clothing for the weather conditions, or access to basic health care). Neglect is tricky because, unlike the situation in the case of divorce, abandonment, or even death, the parent or caretaker is physically present. As a result, the nature of the loss is much harder to detect. For this reason children who suffer from neglect often have a hard time understanding the nature of their suffering. Because their parents or caretakers are physically present, it sometimes is more difficult to recognize the loss. Once again, the result is that children suffer not only from the emotional and functional loss of their parents but also from the added indignity of not having their loss recognized and acknowledged.

Loss of the Sense of Physical Safety

Whether one is battered by a parent, raped by a partner, accidentally shot by a stray bullet in a drive-by shooting, molested by a family member, or beaten during a hate crime, experiences like these deny teens a sense of physical safety. With this loss comes the perception of the world as a dangerous and threatening place. Adolescents who have been physically threatened or brutalized suffer the initial tangible loss that comes with the physical wounds imposed upon their bodies, but worse still is the intangible loss of a sense of safety and trust. After having been physically assaulted, it becomes exceedingly difficult, or traumatic, to let down one's guard, to venture outside of one's narrowly defined zone of comfort, and to risk getting close too others.

Girls, by virtue of their more diminutive stature as compared to boys, are especially vulnerable to being physically assaulted, and hence to the loss of a sense of physical safety. In fact, even when they have never been physically attacked, most girls live with the ominous and ever-present threat that they are easy targets for male aggression, which erodes a sense of physical safety. Similarly, youth who are gay/lesbian/bisexual live with the constant fear of being victimized during a "gay-bashing" incident, which spurs the loss of a sense of safety. Adolescents of color, especially when they are in the presence of police or other "agents of social control" who have a history of unjustly targeting and brutalizing African American and Latino males, also suffer from the loss of a sense of physical safety.

Moving to a New Area

Relocating to a new area can be stressful for a variety of reasons. It's difficult to establish roots in an area that is unfamiliar, and it's hard to relate to people who are complete strangers. The challenge of trying to carve out a little nook for oneself is made all the more difficult by the loss of all that one has left behind. The process of leaving involves the tangible loss of friends, a school, a neighborhood, and a home. Additionally, many teens struggle with the intangible loss of "voice," which is the ability to advocate on one's behalf. Since most parents do not consult with their children about the decision to relocate, their children are left feeling powerless in the decision-making process. Not only must they contend with the physical loss of familiar relationships and community context, but they also must negotiate the loss of any sense of control and personal authority over a significant aspect of their existence.

Loss of Friendship (Not Related to Moving Away)

Adolescence is characterized by an expanding relational network. As young people begin to venture beyond the boundaries of their families, the importance of friendship networks grows dramatically. Because of the salient role that friendships play during adolescence, the loss of one or more friends can be particularly painful. Except in cases where one person moves to another city or state, most friendship losses involve some type of "falling out" between parties. The falling out can occur gradually, as in the case of friends who slowly grow apart as their interests and values change. Or the falling out can occur more abruptly, as in the case of an argument or disagreement that results in two or more friends feeling mutually slighted or offended by each other. The falling out also can be less mutual, as in the case of one friend rejecting another because he or she, for example, refuses to do something that is considered "cool," like smoking or drinking.

Whatever the reason, the loss of a friend is usually very painful for adolescents, who tend to place an extraordinarily high premium on these relationships. Moreover, when a friendship ends because one party has rejected the other, the rejected party must contend not only with the tangible loss of a friend but also with the associated intangible loss of respect, approval, and acceptance that are so critical during this stage of life.

Loss of Diminished Function

In this case, "function" refers to an individual's cognitive, emotional, or physical ability. When one suffers from diminished function, one experiences a loss of one or some combination of their intellectual, emotional, or physical competency. For example, an adolescent may have a learning disability, or may incur an injury that results in some emotional or physical impairment. Regardless of the reason or nature of the specific type of diminished function, the individual experiences a tangible loss of some ability. The difficulty in coping with such a loss is heightened by the associated intangible loss. Most adolescents are extremely self-conscious and concerned about wanting to "fit in" and "be normal." Diminished function threatens a young person's sense of normalcy that often results in a loss of security and confidence. It also can disrupt one's extended community, particularly in cases where athletics are involved. Moreover, if one's peers respond in a rejecting and scornful manner, one is then forced to contend with a loss of peer approval, acceptance, and status, all of which are critical during this stage of development.

Loss of Economic Security

The loss of economic security most commonly arises when parents divorce or a parent loses a job. In either case, a family's socioeconomic status and security can drop substantially. Children and adolescents who were once accustomed to a certain level of material comfort and privilege may suddenly have to adjust to a life of less. When this occurs, there is of course the obvious tangible loss of things like clothes (both in terms of quantity and brand names), accessories and high-tech paraphernalia (ranging from items like cell phones to portable CD players), and opportunities to participate in various social activities (ranging from going to the movies to attending rock concerts and the like). However, with these tangible losses come the intangible loss of peer status and respect, which often is based upon material markers like the types of clothes one wears, the accessories and high-tech paraphernalia one sports, and opportunities to participate in various social activities.

Any number of the losses described above can involve the disruption of community. For instance, moving, separation, divorce, abandonment, and/or death all involve the disruption of community on some level. Therefore, it is important to make the point that disruption of community is synonymous with loss. Individuals who experience a disruption of community have de facto experienced a loss, both tangible and intangible.

The death of Daquon's father was a tangible loss that involved the disruption of his primary community. His father was physically lost to Daquon, but there was an associated emotional and psychological loss as well. With his father's untimely death, Daquon not only lost his father but a piece of himself as well. The bullets that were fired into Daquon's father not only ruptured his spleen but also destroyed Daquon's sense of hope, self-respect, self-worth, and vision for the future.

When his father died, Daquon endured the literal loss of the man he loved and revered, and he also symbolically lost the sense that his own life had meaning and worth. He lost hope for his future. One senseless act of destruction that took less than a second to actualize had consequences that would take Daquon a lifetime to endure. His life was transformed forever. No one-on-one games of hoops, no comforting words for a scraped knee after falling off his bike, no pat on the shoulder after a first outstanding report card. These issues, while seldom discussed, constitute significant losses, especially for a little boy who found himself parentless before he started first grade.

Although Daquon rarely acknowledged it directly, his life was largely encapsulated by hopelessness, despair, and a perpetual sense of yearning. In ways that would be surprising even to him, his bouts with life and living were a daily struggle. He was drawn as though by a magnet toward self-sabotage, self-destruction, and ultimately death—perhaps his morbid way of trying to achieve a sense of community with his parents. If ever there was a physically healthy individual whose life was in need of a social-psychological life preserver, it was Daquon Jackson.

"It was hard growing up without my daddy. I know my grandpops was around, but it wasn't the same as having my daddy. No one could ever take his place. He was a great man, but now no one even knows what a great man he was. Except for me and gramms and grandpops, who even remembers him? Whose gonna remember a black man unless he was a superstar athlete or a superbad criminal? Black men in America die like flies everyday, and no one cares. Hell, I doubt that I will live to 21. It's crazy out there on the streets. If another brother from the hood don't get you, the cops will."

Daquon's haunting words speak volumes about the relationship between loss and devaluation. When his father died, Daquon was confronted with the painful perception that, as a young black male in America, his life was of little value. Unless he became a superhero or a supercriminal, he doubted anyone would even care about his existence. He saw himself as a boy who would never live long enough to be a man. When his father died, Daquon came face to face with the sense of devaluation he felt both as a child without a father and as a young black male in a society whose only use for him was as "target practice."

LIVES THAT ARE BESIEGED BY LOSS

What is especially critical to consider is that, for youth prone to violence, the issue is not just that they have experienced loss but that they have experienced numerous, repeated losses, most of which have never been healed. Loss of any kind is painful, but even more painful than loss itself is when it remains unacknowledged, unmourned, and therefore unhealed. Repeated experiences with unacknowledged, unmourned, and unhealed losses contribute to the dehumanization of loss, which is a precursor to violence. When loss is dehumanized, it is stripped of its meaning. We have found repeatedly that adolescents prone toward violence have a history of losses that have been dehumanized (i.e., unacknowledged, unmourned, unhealed). To cope with the ways in which their losses have been devalued, many adolescents attempt to disconnect themselves from the pain of their losses. Violence is often the anesthetic that they utilize.

Daquon had endured unthinkable losses at a very early age, most of which were unacknowledged, unmourned, and consequently unhealed. The most obvious of his losses was the death of his father. While his grandmother had tried to help him cope with this loss, there were other losses in his life that were virtually unnoticed, unmourned, and unhealed. For example, there was the death of his mother when he was born. According to his grandfather: "Daquon never even knew his mother. You can't miss what you never had." Unfortunately, Mr. Jackson's assessment was not accurate. Even though Daquon had never met his mother, he yearned for her. He yearned for what he believed a mother represented. He saw other children who had their mothers, and he understood the concept of a mother. He also understood that fate had robbed him of the opportunity to know his mother, to experience a fundamental relationship that almost every other child he knew had the chance to experience. If only he could hear her voice calling his name. Being deprived of this opportunity to know his mother and the special bond between a mother and child was a substantial loss. Moreover, the lack of understanding about the loss of his mother prevented those who were closest to Daquon from acknowledging this loss and helping him to engage in a necessary process of mourning and healing.

When Daquon was 8 he was placed in a special education class that separated him from his friends. This was a tangible loss characterized by the disruption of community at the extended level. This also constituted an intangible loss because of the profound devaluation he experienced related to "being put in the class for the stupid kids." This experience was complicated by the fact that Daquon believed one of the reasons he had been placed in a special education class was because he was black. He stated: "I guess they saw me as another dumb nigger, which is why I got put in the retard class. Almost everyone in there was black in a school that had more whites than blacks. So what does that tell you?"

The sense of devaluation he felt as a black person within the context of school assaulted Daquon's sense of community at both the extended level and the cultural level in terms of race. As an African American, he lived with constant assaults to his racial community both within and outside of school, which intensified his feeling of devaluation. Daquon was able to recount numerous experiences in his brief life where he had been the target of racial denigration and discrimination.

Even more significantly, those who devalued Daquon as a black person also devalued his losses, resulting in the dehumanization of loss. For example, after being placed in the special education classroom, Daquon began to act out in class. Unfortunately, his teacher did not seem open to the possibility that maybe his behavior was connected to his placement in this classroom and the loss of respect, dignity, and hope that he had suffered as a result. Consequently, she responded to him punitively rather than compassionately.

THE DEHUMANIZATION OF LOSS

When loss is not acknowledged by others, it loses its meaning—it becomes dehumanized—which is the loss of all losses. Based upon the work we have done in schools, we believe it is highly plausible that one of the reasons why this teacher was unable to recognize and validate Daquon's loss was because she devalued him as a person—as a black person. When a person is devalued, he or she is objectified, stripped of his or her beinghood. It is difficult, perhaps even impossible, to recognize someone's hurt and despair if there is no regard for the essence of their being. If one's beinghood is invisible, then so is his or her pain. Historical and contemporary race relations in the United States provide rich evidence of the ways in which (white) society has consistently objectified black people, thereby devaluing their losses. On more than one occasion, we personally have observed teachers who have ignored the pain and suffering of children of color only to punish them whenever these same children act out their pain in ways that are designed to get someone—anyone—to notice that they exist. It is this subtle but pervasive form of devaluation that ultimately sabotages the healing and resolution of loss.

When loss is dehumanized, healing cannot occur. In Daquon's case, aside from the relatively unsuccessful attempts his grandmother made early on to help him work through the loss of his father, most of Daquon's losses remained unacknowledged, unmourned, and consequently unhealed. Hence, he suffered from the dehumanization of loss. A similar pattern also can be detected in the lives of Carmen and Timothy. The massive disruption of community at all three levels, and the associated devaluation that Carmen endured, were major losses in her life. Her life was besieged with loss, and most significantly little of her loss had ever been acknowledged in a meaningful way. The Brodys were so fearful of addressing the painful experiences in Carmen's life that they conspired to pretend none of it existed. Their denial only bred another layer of loss because, in addition to all that she had endured, Carmen felt devalued by the way her parents pretended that she was just like them and that her life before had not happened.

Certainly, the Brodys' failure to acknowledge the losses in Carmen's life was not the result of a lack of caring about her feelings, but rather because of their deep concern for her. They, like so many others, worried that, by addressing her losses, they would be causing their daughter further pain. Unfortunately, despite the best of intentions, the Brodys only added to Carmen's suffering. By failing to openly acknowledge her losses, Carmen was deprived of the validation she craved for the pain she was feeling. Moreover, because her losses were unacknowledged, Carmen was deprived of the opportunities she desperately needed to mourn and thereby heal the pain she was experiencing. Hence, she too suffered from the dehumanization of loss.

In Timothy's case, his father's abusiveness and what Timothy perceived as his father's abandonment created disruptions in his primary community that left him feeling extremely devalued. Unfortunately, little of this was recognized by his parents—or anyone else, for that matter. Once his father returned and his parents reconciled, they assumed everything was okay. They never thought about how Timothy had suffered a loss, the pain of which still needed to be healed. Since they did not recognize the loss, they could not acknowledge it or help him mourn, which made healing impossible. Moreover, there was virtually no understanding or acknowledgement of the losses Timothy experienced in relation to his class status. It is this reservoir of unacknowledged, unhealed loss, all of which results in the dehumanization of loss, that we believe plays a pivotal role in setting the stage for violence.

CONCLUSION

The dehumanization of loss is strongly tied to devaluation and the disruption of community. Loss is dehumanized when it remains unacknowledged, and therefore unmourned and unhealed. The experience of having one's loss dehumanized is profoundly devaluing. The implicit message is that "My losses haven't been acknowledged because they don't matter . . . because *I* don't matter." Additionally, one of the inevitable consequences of being devalued by others (e.g., family, society) is that one's losses are devalued as well. Hence, for youth who have experienced devaluation, sadly whatever losses they experience more often than not tend also to go unacknowledged, unmourned, and therefore unhealed. Their losses are thereby dehumanized. Finally, because the disruption of community is often experienced as a loss, and because it is a loss that is often tied to devaluation, such disruptions often are not acknowledged, mourned, or healed. All of this underpins the dehumanization of loss that deepens a sense of devaluation and a disruption of community, in an unending downward spiral. In the following chapter we will demonstrate how the complex interaction between these three factors leads to the fourth and final factor in our model—rage—which is the last stop on the path toward violence.

CHAPTER 5

• • • • • • •

Rage

"I hate him! I wish the mothafucker was dead!"

The emotion that radiated from Timothy was pure, undiluted rage.

"Why do you hate him?"

"He's a sissy. He can never defend himself. He always needs Mom or Dad to stick up for him. He is such a little baby. If he wants to mess with me, he's got to face the consequences. All I ever hear is how I have to face the consequences of my actions, so why shouldn't he? If he's too much of a coward to face me, I guess he had better stay out of my way."

Timothy's eyes burned with fury, and he gritted his teeth. His face was contorted by the intense hostility that oozed from him like beads of sweat spilling from open pores on a blistering hot summer day.

According to Timothy's parents, Shaun and Kate, his explosions of rage were increasingly common. The smallest catalyst could set him off. His rage was unpredictable, unstable, and explosive. It was like a live electrical wire thrashing around, hissing, snapping, and whipping through the air, threatening to zap anyone who did not keep his or her distance.

Timothy's latest explosion occurred when his brother, Robert, borrowed one of his CDs without permission. After finding the CD in Robert's player, he went berserk, according to his parents. Timothy's rage turned to violence as he physically assaulted his brother. He pushed him to the ground and kicked him in the stomach. He punched Robert furiously while berating him for taking his CD without permission. When Robert was unable to control his hysterical sobs and cries for help, Timothy began to choke him. Fortunately, their father, Shaun, entered the house from the yard, where he had been working, and heard Timothy screaming, "I'll teach you to shut your fuckin' face and stop whining like a little bitch."

While Timothy's rage appeared entirely dangerous and dysfunctional, it was not the emotion itself that was problematic. Rage is a natural and healthy response to pain and injustice. For adolescents who have experienced devaluation, disruption of community, and unacknowledged loss, rage is inevitable. It is a normal emotional reaction to the pain and suffering that occurs in relation to the other aggravating factors. Rage, in and of itself, is not the problem, but rather the nature of the relationship that adolescents have with it is what is crucial. Adolescents, who are taught to subvert and deny their rage, are deprived of opportunities to learn how to acknowledge and channel it constructively. They also make up the largest group of youth who are most at risk for violence. It is the suppression and denial of rage, as well as the absence of mechanisms for expressing it in positive ways, that increases the probability of violence.

ANGER, RAGE, AND VIOLENCE

When a perceived offense occurs, anger is a common emotional response. Anger arises quickly. It is spontaneous, and if appropriate opportunities exist for the expression and validation of anger, it passes. It has a short life cycle. However, when feelings of anger are suppressed and denied expression or affirmation, they become buried within, eventually taking root and beginning to grow. Suppressed anger is the seed of rage. Over time, suppressed anger grows and intensifies until eventually it is transformed into rage, a far more intense, sustained, and consuming emotion.

When rage is suppressed and limited opportunities exist for healthy expression, it, like anger, grows and intensifies. Over time, the likelihood that suppressed rage will be transformed into violence increases. An essential aspect of preventing violence begins with recognizing rage, finding ways to acknowledge and validate its existence, and encouraging functional opportunities for its expression and release. However, to address rage before it mutates into all-out violence, one must first be able to identify it. At times this can be a challenging endeavor, because rage sometimes manifests itself in ways that make it hard to detect.

DIMENSIONS OF RAGE

Timothy wore the face of *explosive, externally directed rage*. At the slightest provocation he burst into fits of yelling. His eyes would glare, his speech would accelerate, and his muscles would appear tightened as if poised for battle. He was the personification of popular notions of what rage looks like. The manifestation of his rage left little to the imagination in terms of how his rage could be transformed into violence. Those who were witness to the face of Timothy's rage often found it difficult to appreciate the line that divides emotion (rage) from action (violence).

Like Timothy, Daquon carried rage that was prone toward externalization, but, unlike Timothy, Daquon's wasn't the red-faced, burning eyes, loud voice, thrashing fists type of rage. His was a *silent, externally directed rage*. It was a quiet rage that smoldered just beneath the surface of a cold, steely gaze, much like a searing molten lava that burns and bubbles beneath the hardened crust of the earth's surface. The target of Daquon's fury existed outside of himself, but he held his emotion closely in check. The silent nature of his rage often made it difficult for others to realize that Daquon carried an abundance of this emotion within him.

To causal observers, it would almost seem bizarre to characterize Carmen as enraged. Her outward presentation and demeanor didn't match popular notions of "what rage looks like." She never raised her voice or expressed a cruel, cutting word toward anyone. Overall, her affect appeared flat and withdrawn. Clinically speaking, she could have easily been diagnosed as depressed. It is our view that depression is often rage that has been turned inwardly, on the self. Hence, from the perspective of the outside world, the face of Carmen's rage was manifest through what seemed to be pervasive sullenness or depression. She was a textbook example of what we refer to in our work as *internally directed rage*.

THE THREAT OF RAGE

Suppressed rage is the final aggravating factor in our model. It is a precursor to violence. Consequently, we believe that working effectively with violent adolescents requires a proficiency in recognizing and validating rage. This helps to pave the way for helping adolescents develop constructive ways of expressing and channeling their rage. And yet, before any of this is possible, it is necessary to understand some of the obstacles that make it difficult for adults to interact with rage in open, direct, nonreactive ways.

Rage threatens us—or, rather, our anticipation of where rage will lead to threatens us. Our sense of threat is twofold. One aspect involves the threat that rage will expose other strong and more vulnerable emotions like grief, shame, and fear. The other threat is that rage will erupt into violence. Both of these threats make it exceedingly difficult to develop a healthy relationship with rage. Unfortunately, when one has an unhealthy relationship with rage, it makes it almost impossible to deal effectively with the crisis of adolescent violence. Therefore, it is essential to understand the nature of rage, its effects, and how the threats associated with it can be minimized.

RAGE AS A DEFENSE AGAINST MORE VULNERABLE EMOTIONS

Rage can often serve a very sophisticated defensive function for violent and aggressive adolescents. It can operate as a kind of circuit breaker that shuts down one's emotional system before other more vulnerable emotions can be fully experienced. For many youth, the very presence of rage can at times be used to block the expression of more vulnerable emotions such as grief, shame, or fear. To express any emotions of vulnerability, particularly under the "wrong" set of circumstances, can be quite costly within youth culture. After all, to cry or feel lonely, sad, or afraid is to be "soft" in a world that only values being tough. Anger and rage are symbols of toughness—they earn respect. The two personal values that violent and aggressive adolescents hold above all others are to be tough and respected. These are the dynamics that make working effectively with rage and adolescents a major challenge.

The trepidation of having to confront other strong, more vulnerable emotions that tend to underlie rage often contributes to a phenomenon we call "getting stuck in rage." This involves using rage defensively, as a guard against having to feel other feelings. We have heard clients say on countless occasions some variation of the following: "I want to stay mad so I don't have to feel my sadness or hurt." This is why it is so easy and perhaps *preferable* for abandoned children, for instance, to remain angry with their parents than it is for them to embrace their more difficult and vulnerable emotions such as hurt and shame.

The tendency to avoid dealing with vulnerable emotions is not limited to abandoned or violent youth. It is common for virtually all children to absorb and internalize these ways of being. In spite of the verbal messages they receive, they learn through modeling how to become proficient at resorting to rage when they feel hurt, afraid, or ashamed. Boys in particular are socialized to call upon rage whenever other more vulnerable emotions begin to surface. Despite overt warnings against expressions of rage, most boys implicitly learn that because rage is the least vulnerable of strong emotions (and hence the most "manly"), it is one they should call upon when they are at risk of feeling anything else. And, it is precisely because rage is associated with masculinity that girls are strongly discouraged from outward expressions of this emotion.

In the classic film *The Wizard of Oz*, the Wizard appeared to his subjects as a huge, disembodied head immersed in fire that grimaced and frowned, with a voice that roared like thunder. So intimidating was the Wizard that no one had the courage to approach or challenge him. All of the subjects of Oz simply kept their distance, which effectively prevented them from discovering the truth behind the booming voice and the ferocious head. At the end of the film, thanks to the actions of Dorothy's little dog Toto, the curtain is literally pulled back, and the Wizard is exposed for the mere mortal man that he is. In the end, the Wizard was just a person with all the frailties of an ordinary human who simply was doing his best to hide these from the world by projecting a terrifying image. Like the Wizard, many of us use rage as a way of keeping the world at bay. It intimidates others and discourages them from moving close enough to see all that lies beneath the furious front. This is how rage can be used as a defense, as a form of "protection" against the threat of having other, more vulnerable, emotions exposed.

The extreme version of using rage to hide from other emotions can be found in people who are rage-aholics. They are addicted to rage in the same way that an alcoholic is addicted to alcohol. A common denominator unifying all types of addictions is that ultimately, they serve the purpose of helping people to hide from pain, shame, and grief. An addiction numbs a person to her or his emotional agony. Addictions are a form of anesthesia. In the case of a rage-aholic, rage is the poison of choice and the function it serves is to prevent the person from feeling pain.

When rage is used defensively, it is a reaction against a sort of "inner knowing" that, somewhere nearby, a torrent of other strong emotions is lurking. Even when rage is used defensively to try to block these other emotions, there is always the risk that at some point it will burn itself out and all that lies beneath will be exposed. In a society that is as wary of emotion as is ours, is it any wonder than that we respond to rage with trepidation, mistrust, wariness, and even dread?

FROM RAGE TO VIOLENCE

The "threat" that rage poses is not always that it may lead to the release of other more vulnerable emotions. Sometimes it's just the opposite—it's the threat that rage will erupt into violence. The image of rage that lurks in the shadows of our popular imagination is of a person, usually a man, whose entire appearance and demeanor have been distorted by the intensity of this powerful emotion. His temples have become inflated by the protrusion of throbbing veins, his eyes are wide-eyed and burning, the muscles in his face are clenched and contorted, his heartbeat and breathing have accelerated to a frenetic pace, and he's yelling in a voice that blasts the surrounding air like a jackhammer. The threat this man's rage inspires is not so much about the moment itself, but rather of where it will lead. The threat is that expressions of rage will seamlessly mutate into acts of violence. Because of the many times when expressions of rage are indeed a precursor to violence, the two phenomena have become melded in the minds of many.

It is not unreasonable to associate rage with violence. It is in fact one of the reasons why rage occupies such a prominent role in our model of adolescent violence. An indisputable positive correlation exists between the two. Particularly for any one who grew up with a parent or another adult who was prone to fits of rage that crossed over into violence, it is very difficult to appreciate the fine line that separates the two. From the perspectives of those who, as children, were terrorized by raging adults who could also become violent adults, it probably seems like a matter of pointless semantics to draw this distinction. And yet, the distinction is critical.

While rage is often a prelude to violence, this outcome is not inevitable. The two may be closely linked, but they are still two different phenomena. Rage is an emotion. Violence is an action, and the emotion does not always result in the action. In fact, under the right set of circumstances, rage can actually serve as a deterrent to violence.

Whenever we propose the idea that rage can function as a deterrent to violence, we often encounter skepticism from others. Rage and violence are so fused in the minds of many people, that this suggestion defies logic. And yet, we have found repeatedly that *whether rage leads to or away from violence is determined largely by the way in which rage is handled.*

If the response to rage involves a sustained and systematic effort to suppress and/or deny it, this greatly increases the probability that rage will lead to an explosion of violence. The process of suppressing and/or denying rage may create the appearance on the surface that all is calm and secure. But this calm is merely the calm before the storm: it represents anything but security. Suppressing and/or denying rage is like blowing air into a balloon. Like a balloon, rage will expand. Eventually, if rage is suppressed and/or denied long enough, it reaches a bursting point—that fine line where rage, like a balloon that has been inflated beyond its holding capacity, can no longer be contained and will explode. It is this type of explosion that presents the greatest risk of rage being transformed into violence. It is ironic that the motivation for suppressing and/or denying rage arises from a desire to avoid violence. In point of fact, this response has the *opposite* effect: it intensifies rage and the potential for violence.

On the other hand, if the roots of rage are validated and constructive opportunities for channeling and expressing rage are utilized, the likelihood of violence is greatly diminished. For example, youth who find constructive outlets for their rage (athletics, drama, writing, music, sociopolitical activism) are far less likely to become violent because their rage has a channel, and it's a channel that brings them social affirmation, validation, and pride.

Rage is often characterized as irrational, out of control, and destructive, but in fact it is a natural and inevitable response to pain and injustice. It is the emotional culmination of the synergistic interplay between devaluation, disruption of community, and the dehumanization of loss. Individuals who have had experiences with each of these will inevitably experience rage.

When misfortune assaults us, when life lashes out and cruelly taunts and torments us like a schoolyard bully, we encounter pain and a profound, inner sense of injustice. Rage is the fire that gives us the energy, ambition, and determination to survive in spite of our agony. It has weathered millions of years of evolutionary fine-tuning because of the essential role it plays in the survival of our species. When poet Dylan Thomas wrote, "Rage, rage against the dying of the light," he was saying that we must not surrender to injustice, pain, loss, despair, or hopelessness. Instead, we must see the death of hope as a travesty—as life's cruelest injustice—and even against this most despairing and seemingly insurmountable of circumstances, we must resist. Through rage, we must find the inspiration, the will, the raw determination to resist, to never give up, to create hope through never surrendering to hopelessness. Rage is essential to our survival.

In systems that deal in the warehousing of enraged and violent youth (e.g., juvenile detention centers), it can be especially difficult to sell the idea that rage does not automatically equal violence, and in fact, if validated and appropriately channeled, it can actually deter violence. On more than one occasion, we have been told that we "just don't understand." These kids are dangerous. You don't deal with dangerous, violent, criminally inclined kids by allowing them to express rage. Rage is their problem. That's what we're trying to get them to lose. They need to lose the attitudes and check their rage."

Juvenile detention centers and other institutions designed to contain and punish youthful offenders are largely guided by a philosophy that is in opposition to the underlying premise of this book. Systems of this type are not concerned with healing young people. Rather, the primary objective is to detain, punish, and protect society through rehabilitation. Ironically, many of these systems resort to the very tactics they wish to discourage in young people—fear, dominance, and violence as a form of control. As a result, most workers in settings like these are encouraged to use domination and aggression to control youth. Many workers even believe that their own physical survival demands that they respond to enraged youth aggressively, using tactics of domination to suppress expressions of emotion. The unfortunate consequences of such responses to adolescent rage are twofold. First, the rage that so many youth feel is natural and healthy. When systems fail to recognize this and are ill-equipped to deal with rage in constructive ways, they deprive young people of much needed channels for working through and releasing it. This process, unfortunately, intensifies rage rather than diminishing it. Second, the methods that many such institutions employ to suppress rage often are invasive and can intensify devaluation, which ultimately deepens rage.

The way in which these systems are organized makes it very difficult to shift how one thinks about the psychological and social needs of adolescents. It makes it difficult to contemplate the notion that rage does not necessarily equal violence and, in fact, with appropriate guidance and nurturance, it may serve a healing purpose. Those who work in these types of settings and who dare to engage in this type of thinking, by and large, stand alone against the tide. And yet, if those who are the agents of the system can't begin to entertain another vision, let alone another way of doing, what hope does this leave for young people who have even less power and opportunity to transform their conditions? Despite the potentially radical nature of our assertions regarding the anatomy of rage and how to respond to it, we have seen numerous examples of the positive change that is possible when even a single adult is able to relate to an adolescent's rage in ways that move beyond censorship, punishment, repression, and disapproval.

The worry that rage will erupt into violence prevents most of us from appreciating its life-saving power. Consequently, many of us never learn to appreciate that it is not inevitably destructive. A great deal depends on how we interact with rage, how we negotiate it. If we respond to rage by denying and/or suppressing it, or if we channel rage in destructive ways, violence is an almost inevitable conclusion. If however, we are able to acknowledge rage and find constructive channels of expression, the energy that might have otherwise been transformed into violence instead will be converted into a source of healing energy.

UNHEALTHY RELATIONSHIPS WITH RAGE

There is always a history that underpins rage. While anger emerges in the immediacy of a moment, rage builds over time. It is the product of numerous experiences with devaluation, erosion/disruption of community, and the dehumanization of loss that accumulate over time. These are the experiences that sow the seeds of rage. In the following section we pull together the stories of Timothy, Daquon, and Carmen and detail how each of their respective life experiences contributed to their rage and, more specifically, to their unhealthy relationships with their rage. We demonstrate their common experience of never having their rage acknowledged and of never learning how to relate to it positively, while also showing their differences in terms of how they each developed unique ways of manifesting their rage. Ultimately, we illustrate how the synergistic interplay of devaluation, erosion/disruption of community, the dehumanization of loss, and suppressed rage contributed to acts of violence in the lives of each of these young people. In Chapter 10, we outline specific strategies that we employed in each case to assist these teens in constructively rechanneling their rage.

PROFILES OF RAGE

Timothy

"I'm afraid of him. I'm afraid of my own son."

Timothy's mother, Kate, was visibly shaken as she uttered these words. "For years we've had a hard time with him. He's just a difficult kid. I always hoped that one day he'd grow out of it. But this last year or so, he's gotten so much worse. He's always in a bad mood, he lies to us, skips school, he's stolen money out of my wallet, he's started smoking cigarettes. And then, of course, there's the experience with that girl and beating that boy, and now he's hurt his brother, his own brother very badly, all because he used his CD player! I can't even believe he's my son."

Timothy's father, Shaun, interjected: "This is the last straw for us! We have a monster on our hands, and we don't know what to do with him. What he needs is one of those military boot camps where he can learn real discipline and a healthy dose of respect for authority."

Kate added: "We're at our wits' end. Something needs to be done. I just don't understand what's wrong with him. He's so angry all the time. He's filled with hate, and I don't understand why! He hates his brother, I think he hates us; he even hates people he doesn't even know. Sometimes I wonder if it would be better if he were in jail where he couldn't hurt anyone anymore. I just don't trust him, and I have to tell you . . . this is killing me. What kind of mother ever says something like this? It's insane!"

The Ryans were filled with a sense of desperation and confusion. They were convinced that their son was a sociopath, and they felt powerless to reach him and bring him back from the edge of madness on which they saw him teetering.

Timothy sat quietly while his parents spoke. He had heard them rant and rave about him before. There was nothing new here. For years they criticized him for almost everything that he did. He was accustomed to hearing how bad he was, accustomed to being punished for misdeeds that he may or may not have committed. He already knew that his parents thought he was monstrous and that they wanted to get rid of him. And yet, even after hearing it countless times, it still filled him with a deep sense of rage and resentment. It was so unfair that his father had never loved him but that he loved his brother. And it was so unfair the way his mother always blamed him for the problems in the family. These days she often said things like

"You're driving us all crazy—you're the reason we're all falling apart!" Years ago, she was less direct about it, but he knew she blamed him for the time his father had left just by the way she touched him or looked at him. The way she wiped his face after dinner with just enough roughness that he knew she resented him. The way she sometimes got angry when he accidentally spilled milk or splashed too much water during his bath. She was always just a bit on edge, and he knew that in part it was because she couldn't help but think "None of this would be happening if you weren't here."

None of Timothy's fears were true, but through the eyes of a child it all made sense. As a child, he inappropriately personalized his mother's frustration and pain. Her irritability was often unrelated to him, but as a little boy he could not see this, and this is what he remembered. It was what he remembered about his father as well. The routine beatings that Timothy endured at the hands of his father were proof that he was a bad boy who was unworthy of love. Each time a fist landed on his back, his arm, or his chest, he knew it meant his father didn't care about him. Then, during the months that his father was gone, this was the ultimate proof that he was unloved and unwanted. Yet, back then, it didn't stop Timothy from loving and wanting his father in spite of this.

As a little boy, Timothy used to believe in God. He used to pray for his dad to come home. Day after day, he peered out his bedroom window hoping beyond hope that he would see his father coming up the driveway. One day, he heard his mother talking on the phone in the kitchen. She was trying to speak quietly, but Timothy was sitting behind the chair near the doorway. She couldn't see him there. He knew she was talking to his father. He tried to breathe softly so he could hear everything. His mother was saying something about knowing they could work it out and she was trying to give him space. And then she took a big breath and said, "I'm pregnant." According to Timothy, that was the first time he had ever heard that word. He didn't know what it was and was afraid to ask, but he hoped it would bring his dad home.

Timothy prayed again that night. And the next day, he thought it must have worked because his mother seemed happy for the first time in a long time. That's when he found out what the strange word meant. Timothy recalled his mother saying the following: "Timothy, I have something wonderful to tell you. I'm pregnant, honey. That means I'm going to have a baby. You're going to have a little brother or sister. And the best part is, I talked to your dad last night, and I really think things may work out. I don't want to get your hopes up yet, but I really have a good feeling."

Timothy couldn't remember another time in his life when his mother seemed so happy. "Her face lit up like a full moon . . . I mean, she was beaming!" he stated. But Timothy was feeling something altogether different. The hope he'd felt when he first saw his mother that morning was washed over by a cloud of confusion and doubt. What did that mean he was "going to have little brother or sister"? And why was this the one thing that was going to bring his dad home? Why was his dad willing to come back for the little brother or sister that no one even knew yet, but he hadn't come back for Timothy? The more he thought about it, the more saddened and then angry he became. "It wasn't fair." Timothy uttered angrily: "The bastard didn't love me enough to come back for me, but he was willing to come home for a son he had never even met before."

What Timothy never realized, of course, was that the timing between his father's return and his soon-to-arrive new baby brother was not nearly as related as he thought. According to Shaun, the timing of his return was more a matter of economics than a preference for one child over another. He had finally gotten a secure job, and, as a result, for the first time in a long time he felt prepared to assume his role as provider, husband, and father. In therapy sessions, he repeatedly tried to assure us, as well as his family, that "it was never the way Timothy had imagined it in his head." But it didn't matter, because Timothy believed it happened the way he remembers it. And as a result, both Shaun and his relationship with his son have suffered in the same way it would have if it had been exactly the way Timothy remembers it. Unfortunately, Shaun has been unable to see how or why Timothy could see it the way he does. Timothy, on the other hand, is enraged with his father because "he won't be man enough to just admit things."

After his dad came home, Timothy hoped he would see some sign of his father's love. He didn't. During the first few months of his dad's return home, Timothy was still subjected to routine beatings. He could still recall the feeling of utter powerlessness whenever his father pushed him down or twisted his arm. He felt intense fear and pain, but, somewhere even deeper down, he felt rage. He was furious with his father for hurting him, but he was even more furious with himself for not being big enough and strong enough to protect himself. He resented his own helplessness.

Shortly after Robert's birth, Shaun became less and less physically aggressive with Timothy until eventually this behavior was all but a thing of the past. But for Timothy, his memories of those experiences never faded. They remained as vivid as if they had happened just yesterday.

From the time he was a little boy, Timothy had lived with the pain of feeling unloved and unwanted, the ultimate form of devaluation. In response to the pain of his loss (of love, nurturance, affirmation), he felt deep rage. Robert never had to do much of anything to incite Timothy's rage; his existence was a form of incitement. In Timothy's eyes, his brother symbolized his devastating loss, the loss of the father and the love he so desperately craved. Timothy was full of rage. He was furious with his father and brother; he was furious with his father for rejecting him and his brother for having "stolen the love" that he so desperately wanted and felt entitled to as the first-born son. Of course, most of Timothy's rage was directed at his brother rather than his father, because Robert was younger, smaller, and weaker—an easier target. But also Timothy understood on some level that by "getting" his brother, he was indirectly "getting at" his father and punishing him for the rejection he had felt since he was a small boy.

The fact that Timothy's parents were mystified by his behavior was symptomatic of the issues with which he was struggling. Kate and Shaun were both committed parents, and they were doing the very best job they could with their children. They had overcome major obstacles in their marriage and had worked hard to hold their family together. Unfortunately, however, they never noticed the effects that their problems had on little Timothy. He was only a small boy when they were struggling through the most difficult years of their marriage. Certainly it doesn't make them bad parents; in fact, we would say they were good parents in many important ways. But the stress in their lives was so overwhelming that it made it hard for them to see just how deeply their son was being affected by the chaos, uncertainty, and disruption around him. Moreover, they made the same mistake that many parents make. They assumed that, once they were on steadier ground, their children would naturally follow suit.

For Timothy, however, who had lived through a period of great turmoil and had suffered damaging blows to his self-esteem, he was carrying around unhealed trauma wounds that had never even been acknowledged by his family. The abuse he was subjected to as a young child had deeply wounded him emotionally. Moreover, the day Shaun moved out, Timothy felt as if he had lost his father, and hence his sense of family, of community at the primary level, was irrevocability shaken. The blow to his self-esteem was devastating. Timothy incurred a deep, profound sense of devaluation. These wounds were exacerbated by Robert's birth, because in Timothy's mind Robert became the symbol for the love he believed he had lost. Every time Timothy looked at Robert, he felt the pain of what he perceived as the loss of his father's love, the loss of the sense of family he yearned for, for the validation of his essential worth and *loveableness*. In response to all of this, Timothy experienced a deep sense of rage.

Because his parents did not see or understand the nature of Timothy's suffering, they were never able to validate his pain and help him heal his wounds. This lack of validation for Timothy's pain exacerbated his sense of devaluation, reinforced his feeling of being alienated from the secure bosom of a family, intensified his sense of loss, and magnified his sense of rage. With each passing day, he became more and more agitated, snappy, and embittered. Unfortunately, rather than recognizing his rage as a signal of underlying pain, and helping him to address it and the underlying wounds, he was simply punished further, intensifying the entire vicious cycle. It was only now that Timothy's explosive rage was reaching a crisis point and rapidly mutating into full-fledged acts of violence that, at last, he and his family would begin the process of saving both Timothy and themselves.

Daquon

"I wanted him to hurt for what he did. What he did was wrong, and he needed to pay for what he did." Daquon's words were intense, but his emotion was flat. He was talking about revenge for a horrible crime. He was speaking about retribution and retaliation against a heinous act, the murder of a friend. The death of Big G was a travesty. He'd been shot to death in front of his mother's house. Big G had just returned from the store and was dropping off the items his mother had requested. According to Daquon, "Big G never saw this coming . . . he never even had a chance." His death came spinning around the corner in a car from which the deadly shots were fired into his back. The groceries he carried only moments earlier were now splattered on the pavement, the cold milk mixing with his warm blood in a puddle of madness. The police determined that the crime was unsolvable and recorded it as another Southside homicide. There were more of those in a week than anyone cared to count.

"He was my homeboy. We had each other's backs. Been that way since we were 10. No one smokes my blood that doesn't have to face me. Big G would have done the same for me." Daquon was talking about friendship, brotherhood, and loyalty. He and Big G shared a deep bond, and when Big G was murdered, the loss ripped through Daquon's soul the same as if G had been his biological brother. Daquon had been through his once before, when his father was fatally shot before his very eyes when he was only 5. And, of course, he was reminded of it every time he heard about another brother from the hood—someone like him, like G, like his dad—who'd been killed. But, no, he had not grown used to it. No matter how many times Daquon had lived the terrors of life in a war zone, he had never grown accustomed to the sight of a loved one lying lifeless and mutilated on a sidewalk. He had not grown used to seeing their blood gush from their bodies, taking with it the love he wanted and needed.

Looking at Daquon as he made his veiled reference to his intended retribution, it was frightening how calm and cool he appeared. There were no signs of the irrational, out-of-control rage that one might have expected. His face was as expressionless as a stone, and his eyes seemed cold and impenetrable, but there was an intensity that immersed him that seemed to suck up all the air in the room. In contrast to Timothy's explosive, volatile rage, Daquon exuded a hushed, silent rage that was deceptively quiet but undeniably present.

Just looking at Daquon, without any prior knowledge of him, it would be easy to fear him. Despite his outward appearance of composure, one immediately felt "on guard" in his presence. He never had to say a word; he didn't need to shout, raise a fist, or show any other outward sign of aggression. His very presence carried an unspoken threat. Sitting in the confines of the eight-foot-by-eight-foot cube known as a "therapy room," it was impossible not to feel this threat, not to feel his rage and the lethality that its intensity implied. It was difficult not to be distracted by it. His presence was so discomforting that instinctively one wanted to distance oneself from him, to move away from the energy he emitted. And most people did move away from him—or they tried to control him, to contain his energy field, to suppress or better yet, extinguish it.

Daquon had spent the past 4 months in a "youth center," which was merely a euphemistic phrase for a juvenile penitentiary. The official charge was stealing, which resulted in the revocation of his probation associated with a prior conviction for stealing. More accurately, however, the "crime" leading to his latest incarceration was his rage.

Daquon seemed to make Mrs. Fleishman, the teacher who had filed the charge, uncomfortable. She was afraid of him. His very presence appeared to make her jittery. As far as Daquon was concerned, when she had the opportunity to get rid of him, she grabbed it. Daquon knew that any one of the 28 students in the class could easily have taken her wallet. Everyone knew where she kept it, and it would have taken only a second or two to ease the drawer open and slip the wallet out. In this instance, the wallet was lying on her desk, making its theft all the easier.

When Mrs. Fleishman realized the wallet was gone, it seemed that each little bit of circumstantial evidence melded in her mind to convince her that Daquon was the guilty party. As she had reported, "I know the wallet was on my desk before the class entered the room. I only stepped away from my desk briefly to consult with another student. I saw Daquon near my desk during that time, and he has been known to do this type of thing." Of course, it is very likely that the most convincing evidence of all—the piece of evidence that Mrs. Fleishman seemed most oblivious to—was her evident discomfort with and possible disliking of Daquon. She may very well have been unnerved by Daquon's unsmiling demeanor, his steely gaze, his looming stature, and of course the fact that he was a young black male.

Daquon had been passing through the halls on his way to English class, the only class he actually liked in school. He was looking forward to class that day because his teacher, Mrs. Green, was returning the latest composition, on which he had worked hard. He was excited about the topic, "The Significance of Richard Wright's *Native Son* for Young Black Males in the 1990s." He just knew he would get an "A." But he never it made it to class that day. He saw the two officers, escorted by the principal, approaching from the other end of the hallway. At first he didn't know it was him they were coming for, but nonetheless his gut tightened. He always felt a moment of anxiety when he saw the police.

When he saw the principal point in his direction, he realized soon enough that it was him they were coming to get. He couldn't imagine what the problem was; after all, he had been keeping to his own business. It wasn't like he was hanging out on a street corner or walking through a store—places where he might expect to be identified as a menace. But in his heart he knew better. As a young black male, it didn't matter where he was or what he was doing. Yet, Daquon never gave them the satisfaction of losing his cool. He never let them see it get to him. They cuffed him in the middle of the hall and "escorted" him out to the squad car, with half the student body looking on in amusement.

Within days after his arrest his probation was revoked, and Daquon was back in the youth center completing the remainder of his 6-month sentence for a prior conviction for stealing. Returning to the center 8 months after he had left was like watching a rerun of a bad movie. He just hoped the time would go quickly. While he would never let anyone know it, he hated small, confined spaces.

Daquon had been in the youth center for 2 months when Big G was shot and killed. His grandmother came the very next day to tell him. "I felt like someone had slammed a steel pipe into my ribs," Daquon recalled. He said that his first thought was of the last time he had seen Big G. It was the day before he had been arrested at school. They had made plans to get together over the weekend and watch the Raiders/Cowboys game. Daquon was a diehard Raiders fan, and Big G had been devoted to the Cowboys since he was a little boy. "Man, you know the Cowboys will whup the Raiders' asses. You just hanging onto a pipe dream thinking your boys is gonna come through for you . . . finally." Big G laughed, delighted with himself for his teasing jab.

Daquon laughed, too. "Okay, Money, we'll see who's laughing come Sunday when the Raiders dog your little Cowgirls." Daquon was pleased with his jab back. The two boys were well versed in this back-and-forth game of verbal combat—they'd been engaged in it for years. It was a sign of deep affection.

Daquon could still see Big G smiling as he scooped up his jacket and headed for the door to leave. If only Daquon had known it was the last time he would ever see his friend. He would have said the one thing that both boys were only able to say to each other once, while under the influence of several beers (meaning it didn't really count because liquor made folks do crazy things they couldn't be held responsible for): "I love you, man." If only it hadn't been so hard to say. They both knew it was true, but each had been bound by the code of male honor that said "real men" didn't identify with the type of open affection and sweet emotion more characteristic of the "weaker" sex—females. But while neither dared break with the code, they both felt their mutual affection to be as strong and as deep as if they had been born brothers. They loved each other, and although they both knew it, Daquon wished he had been able to say it to G directly.

Day after day, sitting alone, feeling as if the walls were closing in on him, Daquon thought about G, and he thought about the way he died. The more he thought, the more intensely furious he felt. He saw his friend walking down the street, imagined the car with the hit man in it spinning around the block. He could see the bullets, as if in slow motion, slicing through the air and landing in Big G's back. He saw them rip through his flesh and lodge themselves in the cavity of his body, the blood gushing out of his wounds as his body crumbled to the ground, never again to rise. He saw the car with G's executioner in it disappearing down the street, never to be called to justice. Daquon felt his insides burn with rage. The heat of his rage was so intense that many nights it kept him awake. He lay in his bed staring at the ceiling, and all he could do to comfort himself was imagine how, when he was out, he would somehow track down those who were responsible and do to them what the law would not do: make them pay.

Daquon spent his daytime hours in the center keeping busy with whatever he was required to do. He had a reason to get out of the center as soon as possible, so it was critical that he kept himself together. But that was easy enough; he had lots of practice with looking low-key. He'd learned long ago how to never let his thoughts or feelings show outwardly. As a black male, his survival depended upon his learning this lesson. Daquon, like many young black males, had learned what Majors and Mancini-Billson (1992) have referred to as the art of "cool posing," which is a form of posturing that enables black males to project an air of poise under pressure. No matter how challenging, unsettling, or threatening external conditions may be, one assumes an almost aloof "nothing-can-faze-me" stance. Cool posing is a way of looking adversity or possible humiliation in the eye and mocking it. It is a way of "never letting them see you sweat."

While speculations abound regarding the roots of cool posing, there is little doubt that it plays an essential role in the lives of contemporary black males. At the very least, it allows black males to "save face" when confronted with the almost daily indignities that assault them in a racist society. More importantly, cool posing plays a crucial role in the politics of survival. As in Daquon's case, when one must live with his back almost always pressed up against a wall, it is critical to learn how to maintain one's cool—to never let the aggressor taste the scent of blood, so to speak. Almost all people who live their lives on the margin develop strategies for shielding their inner life and emotions from their oppressors' direct gaze. Daquon was a master of the cool pose. The world around him could be completely up in arms, but he never flinched. To the naked eye, his flawless air of cool, his unfettered calm, the perfect sense of masculine bravado that was implied in his almost defiant physical posture, made him seem impenetrable. There was something decidedly intimidating about his demeanor. It was unnerving to observe his unflappable front—it was hard not to believe all that it implied, hard to keep in mind that somewhere underneath it all there was an ordinary human being, a kid who had been hurt in ways that were unimaginable, a boy who felt rage, pain, grief, and even fear. We tried to bear this in mind as we sat across from him during our first session following his release from the youth center only days before.

Daquon had been a model of good behavior in the center (undoubtedly a direct benefit of his cool posing skills), so he was released early. One of the terms of his release was that he had to attend therapy. Given our prior relationship, we were a natural choice as the therapists who were to work with him during his probationary period. It was helpful that we were already well acquainted with him, and we sensed that Daquon trusted us. We had gained his respect when we first worked with him during the 3 months prior to his second stint at the youth center. It also seemed to have been important to him that we remained in contact with him during his lockup time.

He came to the session in his usual street duds: baggy jeans, unlaced Timberland boots, and hooded red sweatshirt. Because we had already earned his trust, he freely discussed the events that had led up to his return to the youth center, and he described without hesitation the circumstances surrounding Big G's untimely death. He even went so far as to admit that he would see justice done by his friend, whatever it took. Looking into his unflinching gaze, we believed that he meant what he said. He possessed a sense of chilling resolve about what he would have to do. And while there were no obvious external clues to alert us to the fact that Daquon was consumed with rage, it was there in the room, just beneath his cool facade, burning his insides and silently sucking up the air in the small therapy room. While Daquon was no less enraged than Timothy, the silent nature of his rage created the illusion that he was less distressed. Those less attuned to Daquon's life story and psychology, on observing his demeanor, might be shocked by the moment when, without warning and with deadly precision, he would suddenly lash out. Because we were observing him not only with our eyes but also with our hearts and intuition, we saw what lay beneath Daquon's steely gaze and stony expression. We saw the rage beneath the front and the pain behind the rage, and we knew we needed to move quickly to deal with both before they erupted into an episode of violence. It was a race against time.

Carmen

"I wasn't trying to kill myself. I just had too much to drink and I passed out." The "too much" that Carmen was referring to culminated with her being rushed to the hospital emergency room, where she was diagnosed with alcohol poisoning. She had consumed so much vodka that her entire system was on the verge of shutting down permanently.

A resident advisor found her passed out in the bathroom of her dormitory. The bottle of vodka she had nearly finished—probably not her first of the night—was still clenched tightly in her fist. After she arrived at the emergency room, a trauma team worked on her for several hours, miraculously pulling her back from the brink of death.

She sat before us looking frail and small. Her shiny black hair was hanging listlessly around her face. She had dark, purplish-black circles under her eyes, and her normally honey-brown complexion looked deadened and sallow.

"How do you feel about the fact that you might have died, even though, as you say, that was not your goal?"

There was a long silence. She twisted slowly, almost painfully, in her chair. Her gaze shifted inward, as if she were trying to disappear from view.

"I don't know," she finally answered. "It probably wouldn't make that much difference."

"Why is that?" we asked.

"Nothing seems to matter too much these days."

To the casual observer, it would almost seem bizarre to characterize Carmen as enraged, because her outward presentation didn't match popular notions regarding "what rage looks like." Overall, her affect appeared flat and withdrawn. Clinically speaking, she could easily have been diagnosed as depressed. Hence, from the perspective of the outside world, the face of Carmen's rage was manifest through what seemed to be pervasive sullenness or depression.

To look at Carmen was to see a girl who seemed emotionally barren and devoid of all hope. It was hard to imagine what could leave someone so young-looking so defeated. Certainly there were her horrific early childhood experiences—the trauma of losing her parents and the terror and loneliness she felt during her months in the orphanage. Here also was the massive disruption and fear she felt when she was adopted by the Brodys and forced to leave behind the only life she had ever known in rural Peru. Her new life meant moving thousands of miles from home and living with a family she did not know in one of the world's largest cities. The disruption and loss Carmen endured before she was even 8 years old would be hard for even the worldliest adult to imagine. And of course, in addition to adapting to life with a new family, there were her struggles to adjust to her new environment in terms of her national, racial, class, linguistic, and religious identification.

Even after Carmen began to trust the Brodys and ease into the security of their embrace, she continued to feel the emptiness of being an outsider in a nation that would never be her own. She lived with the constant ache of knowing that every part of the world she had left behind, and every part of who she was deep within, was unacceptable in her new world. To the "gringos" (as she sometimes called here detractors in rare uncensored moments), no matter how flawlessly she spoke English (she had lost her accent long ago) or what private prep schools or Ivy League university her parents paid her way through, she was still only half of a human being in their eyes. She was just an Indian from the primitive, savage "jungles" of South America (even if she had never seen a jungle in her life).

But while all of this was deeply painful, those who loved her most would have argued strongly that Carmen had healed her pain over the last 10 years. They would have pointed out that the most traumatic years of her life were long behind her. There was evidence to suggest she had adjusted well to her new life, and was in fact thriving. The pictures in the family photo album revealed a girl who smiled a lot and who was surrounded by people who loved her—there were so many happy-looking times. And, despite a difficult initial adjustment period, Carmen became one of the top students in her school, receiving straight A's. Certainly she was quiet and tended to be introspective, but how could anyone doubt that she had been happy for the last 10 years? Given all she had survived, and in light of the seeming happiness and transformation during the past decade, it seemed hard to understand how Carmen had spiraled to the edge of such despair. It seemed even harder to imagine that she was feeling anything that could approximate rage.

•　•　•　•

Carmen couldn't help staring at Kent—he was definitely beautiful in a classically Grecian sort of way. Each and every muscle rippled with statue-like perfection. Carmen would never forget the day she first laid eyes on him. He was wearing a sky-blue tank top that showcased his Adonis-like torso, and his flaxen hair glistened in the noonday sun. He was standing on the marble steps leading up to the library, and while sitting on a bench under a tree across the lawn from him, she was able to watch him inconspicuously.

It never occurred to Carmen that Kent would ever notice her or have any interest in her, so when he started pursuing her for a date, she was overcome with giddy delight. Their first date was magical to Carmen, and happily it led to many more. Kent seemed to adore her. He told her she was like an exotic flower. He had never dated an Indian before, and he seemed to find her dark beauty mysterious and mesmerizing. Carmen wasn't sure she was completely comfortable with the way he exoticized her. There was something about it that made her feel a bit inhuman, but it seemed to be in a good way. After all, Kent was extolling her beauty and he seemed to cherish her like a precious treasure, so what could be the problem in that?

Carmen and Kent dated seriously for 4 months. He was her first serious boyfriend, and she was delighted to finally have one, especially someone as wonderful as Kent. But then, just 1 day before returning to school for the new semester, it all came apart. Kent called her at home to break up with her. He had met someone new and professed that he was "in love." Carmen was in shock. She could not make sense of the words she was hearing. How, after everything they had shared, could he be saying something so foreign, so cold, to her? She cried into her pillow all night long, and the next day when her mother asked her why her eyes were puffy, she lied.

Back at school Carmen was tortured every time she saw Kent with his new love, Sandy. She was everything that an all-American boy's dreams were made of. She was tall and leggy, with an ample bosom and curvaceous hips. She had a long golden mane of hair that sashayed when she walked, and sparkled almost as much as her pale blue eyes. Even as she walked across the lawn with Kent glued to her side, men's heads turned to stare at her. She was stunning. In fact, she was the one thing Carmen could never be—she was white. Even if Carmen dyed her hair, worked out in the gym every day, got breast implants, and wore contact lenses, she could never be as perfect as Sandy. While Sandy was striking in many ways, above all else it was her smooth white skin—even while it had been ever so slightly bronzed by the sun—that made her flawless in Carmen's eyes. To Carmen, she had not been dumped for just another woman—she had been dumped for a *beautiful white woman*.

Comparing herself to Sandy, Carmen plunged into an abyss of self-hatred whose true depths she had not fully recognized until that very moment. It threw her back into Mrs. Peabody's fifth-grade math class, where she obsessed about Christie Tyler's strawberry-blond locks. She had so much yearned to touch Christie's hair, to possess it, rip it out by the roots, and transplant in into her own head. And how she yearned for that snow white skin with the honey-colored freckles that looked as if they had been painted on Christie's perfectly round little nose. Mostly she yearned not to be the only child in her class with the dark, stained complexion and the black eyes. Oh, how she hated the way she looked, the way it made her different—different in a way that she knew was ugly and shameful. She knew it because every time she opened her sister's *Seventeen* magazine and *YM* she never saw herself reflected there. All she ever saw were girls like Christie and Sandy. And she knew it because every time her parents took her some place "good," where smart, beautiful, elegant people were—like the ballet, the opera, the summer vacations in Pebble Beach and West Palm, and the ski trips to Vail and Aspen—in all these places, she never saw anyone who looked like her. She saw Christies and Sandys, but never anyone like herself.

The only time Carmen remembered seeing people like herself was in Taos, New Mexico. She first saw them at the roadside stands, selling woven baskets and turquoise jewelry. She recalled feeling relieved to finally see people who looked like her. In her heart, Carmen felt a connection for the first time since she had left Peru. She felt a yearning that she had buried long ago. The people she saw, although strangers, were more familiar to her than her friends back in New York. And when she looked into their eyes, she saw home, but she also saw pain and suffering. When she asked her mother for thirty dollars for the pair of sterling silver and turquoise earrings, her mother replied: "That's too much. You can't trust these people here, because they'll try to rob you. I'll get you something nice later." When she heard these words from her mother, they were words she would never forget—and perhaps never forgive.

Her mother could have meant anything by "these people," but Carmen knew what she meant. Her mother didn't trust them because they were poor and Indian. They were also Carmen, her daughter, but her mother couldn't see that now. She couldn't see that her own daughter was the person she did not trust. Somehow, Carmen's Indianness and the poverty she had been born into were invisible to her mother. But Carmen could see it, and in her heart she knew it meant she would never be as real a person—as real a woman—as someone like Sandy. She would never be as valuable, no one would ever love and want her as much as she needed to be loved and wanted. And if by chance someone, someday did, it could only be because they were more flawed than she.

For the next several weeks after Kent broke up with her, Carmen tried to keep herself busy, but she was caught up in a difficult cycle of sleeping too much or not enough. At times, she was unable to sleep or calm herself, she would study for hours and hours. Then she would crash and plunge into a deep sleep, unable to wake herself or get out of bed. She missed several classes as a result, but made up for it with the marathon study sessions that always followed during her sleepless stretches. Because of her erratic lifestyle and the obvious strain on her health, and because she was never very regular with her periods, Carmen had not noticed that she hadn't had a period since last semester. In fact, she had missed most of the obvious warning signs until a doctor finally diagnosed her one day after she had collapsed while walking to class and was taken to the health center.

She was pregnant. At first she was terrified, then excited. She thought it might mean something wonderful to Kent, but she was wrong. When she first met with him to tell him, he misinterpreted her call as an invitation to reopen their sexual relationship. Carmen was stunned, confused, and offended. Nonetheless, she held her ground and told him about the pregnancy. He was furious and he accused her of trying to trap him with a child that was not his. She insisted that it was, and finally he lunged at her, grabbing her by the throat. The following is how Carmen reported the conversation to us as she spoke in a whisper-like tone:

> KENT: Listen to me, you little tramp. I'm no fool. You can't fuck me over with this little game. I finally have everything I want, and you're not going to destroy it all. Do you honestly believe I would have a little nigger baby with you? DO YOU?! Get real!
>
> CARMEN: I am sorry . . . I am really sorry

After several minutes of silence and Carmen crying incessantly, she reported that he told her:

> KENT: Carmen I'm sorry. I didn't mean to hurt you. I never wanted to hurt you. And I'm sorry you're pregnant. But you can't keep

this child. Look, I'll pay for the abortion. Okay? I'll even find out where you can get it done. You won't have to worry about anything.

According to Carmen, "He said a few more things, but I was only half hearing him. His voice seemed so distant. I think at this point I just retreated into an inner world where he could not touch me. It was a place deep inside, a place I had been to once before in my life, when I was around 7."

Days later Carmen had an abortion. Her friends tried to comfort her. They encouraged her to be angry with Kent, but Carmen excused him and blamed herself. She later felt that some of her friends became angry and frustrated with her because of her lack of anger toward Kent.

What her friends failed to realize was that Carmen was pissed. She did have rage, but it was difficult to detect. Even she, Carmen, would not have described herself as enraged. It was an emotion she would not allow herself to acknowledge, which was one of the reasons she had so much of it. There were many reasons her rage remained so deeply buried, so masked behind depression and sullenness. Her gender socialization was probably a major reason. As a girl she was inclined toward the internalization of rage. She bought into the "good girls don't get angry" hype. She embodied the demure, slightly deferential stance of a "nice girl" who was on her way to becoming a "decent woman." While no one had ever told her outright she should bury her own inner desires, passions, and opinions, she (like most girls) learned that, if she was to become a good woman, this was exactly what she would have to do. In a thousand ways each day of her life, she was shaped and molded by a culture that demands, as the price for its patriarchal fortification, the spirits, minds, and hearts of its female children. As Mary Pipher (1994) described in her book *Reviving Ophelia: Saving the Selves of Adolescent Girls*, the transition from girlhood to womanhood involves the surrendering of girls' voices, of their personal authority, and of their inner knowing, fire, and dynamism. Carmen was no exception. In fact, as a child of color lost in a sea of whiteness, she was even more prone to the conditioning process that left her feeling unentitled to her opinions or her feelings. As a girl who was becoming a woman, and as a person of color in a white world, she already had mastered how to artfully suppress, contain, constrain, and deny her own thoughts and emotions, even to the point that she became unknown to herself. She had learned the art of agreeability, passivity, compliance, and of course blankness—an expression of nothingness that connotes an absence of presence, memory, or will.

According to Carmen, "the rest of the semester was a blur." She shifted in and out of her inner and outer worlds, and because she needed more than ever to be a good girl, she somehow managed to get through all her classes with decent grades: one A–, four B's. For anyone who bothered to notice, she appeared sad and withdrawn. But no one noticed. No one saw the shame and humiliation, her self-loathing, her inner tears, or, for that matter, her rage. That was one thing even she herself did not see, because, above all else, good girls did not display an emotion as vile, ugly, and as boorishly masculine as rage.

Over the summer break Carmen was introduced to alcohol by several well-meaning friends who wanted to party. In time, she realized she could use alcohol to distance herself, at least temporarily, from her pain. By the time she returned to school in the fall, she was accustomed to drinking herself to sleep almost every night. Several weeks into the semester a resident advisor found her almost dead in the bathroom. After narrowly escaping death, a week later she was sitting across from us in our therapy office.

In spite of the fact that popular characterizations of rage made it difficult to detect Carmen's, there was little doubt of the cauldron of rage that resided deep within her. The challenge in her case was not just in bringing the rage to the surface where others could bear witness to it, but in helping even Carmen to see it. She was so disconnected from her own pain, so convinced she did not have a right to her suffering or her rage, that she could not allow herself to see herself clearly. Hence, our work with her had to begin with a journey toward helping her reclaim her lost parts, including her rage, which would naturally give way to the process of helping Carmen rechannel and deal with the rage more constructively.

CONCLUSION

While Timothy, Daquon, and Carmen all "wore" their rage in different ways, each of them had an unhealthy relationship with their rage. The rage of Timothy and Daquon was externally directed. However, Timothy's rage was much more explosive than Daquon's, who manifested his rage quietly, with a chilling sense of control. Carmen's rage, in contrast, was so deeply buried and inwardly focused that it was undetectable to the naked eye. But, in spite of these differences, each one was filled with rage. None of them had ever had their rage validated or had learned healthy ways of channeling it; consequently, they were each a prime candidate for the transformation of rage to violence. Already, Timothy had physically assaulted his brother and his parents feared—rightfully so—that without intervention it was only a matter of time before he did worse. Daquon was plotting revenge for the murder of his best friend, and nothing less than "an eye for an eye" would do. He had spent months fantasizing about and plotting his moment of violent retribution. Carmen had turned inwardly and was slowly poisoning herself to death. Day after day she had been pouring toxic levels of alcohol down her throat, rapidly hurling herself to the edge of self-destruction. It was only by a miracle that she had not already succeeded in killing or permanently injuring herself. Her rage, like that of Daquon and Timothy, already had mutated into violence, and without immediate intervention, destruction was inevitable. All three of them desperately needed help. All three of them were literally dying to be saved.

PART II

· · · · · · · ·

Strategies

CHAPTER 6

• • • • • • •

Adolescent Axioms
General Principles
for Working with Adolescents

Many adults generally struggle with how to understand and relate to most teens, even those who are not violent. When an emotionally volatile issue like violence is factored into the equation, this only intensifies anxiety. Hence, we believe a brief discussion about working with adolescents in general is necessary before discussing violent adolescents. In our view, the work we do with adolescents who show some tendencies toward violence and aggression is an outgrowth of a set of baseline beliefs we hold regarding working with adolescents in general.

Our early work with adolescents, even in the most benign cases, was often fraught with anxiety, complications, and ultimately lots of mistakes. Our good intentions, no matter how well thought out or carefully executed, seldom rendered the results we wanted. It seemed virtually inevitable that we would say the wrong thing, do the wrong thing, do too much of this or not enough of that in most of our interactions with the adolescents with whom we worked. Our numerous well-intentioned but failed attempts "to connect with them" often resulted in one or both of us becoming more and more controlling. Predictably, the more we tightened the reins and made more authority-laced demands, the more they rebelled. The more they resisted and rebelled, the more we demanded and attempted to control, even in the face of compelling data indicating that our approach was not delivering the results we desired.

Over the years we have gleaned a number of valuable lessons from our work with adolescents. Most of these lessons, as we are suggesting here, were learned the hard way, whether it was through trying to force a willfully silent teen to speak or attempting to engage a typically skeptical youth with our "I'm cool" posturing. All of these experiences have resulted in a set of axioms that we use to guide our work with adolescents today. We often refer to these as our "adolescent axioms." Since employing these, we have experienced a welcomed and dramatic shift in our work. While not a panacea, they have assisted us in thinking differently about adolescents and the nature of the work we do with them. No, the axioms have not entirely eliminated the rough spots, but they have helped a great deal. Our work nowadays is beset far less by the power struggles that too often characterized it during the early going. Embracing these axioms has helped us to step outside of our egos in regard to our work. We seem to have a better handle on the shortsightedness of viewing so much of what adolescents do as a personal affront to us as professionals and adults. We see the axioms, while obviously not intervention strategies in the purest sense, as a framework that helps us develop the type of approach with adolescents that makes effective and substantive work possible.

ADOLESCENT AXIOMS

1. Expect Madness, Badness, and No Easy Rides

From the perspectives of most adults, adolescents often exhibit bizarre vacillations between states of childlike innocence and adult sophistication—hence, a form of madness. Trapped somewhere between childhood and adulthood, adolescents frequently struggle to mediate their conflicting needs and desires. On the one hand, they crave to be free, independent, and self-sufficient young adults. On the other hand, they long for the safety and security typically associated with the world of childhood. The pressure and uncertainty that these competing needs create often lead to behaviors that seem quite maddening to adults. At other times, the rebellious, reckless actions of adolescents are what many adults describe as teen "badness." Premarital sex, drinking, smoking, and deafening blasts of music are behaviors that are viewed as indications that a once sweet, lovable child has become a hellion. Whether it's madness or badness, the bottom line for those of us interacting with adolescents is to understand that "there are no easy rides." In most cases, some type or degree of hassle is inevitable.

The complexities, ambiguities, and apparent contradictions associated with teen madness were highlighted for us just the other day when we spoke with Mr. Mateo, an exasperated and bewildered parent. He was describing the seemingly bizarre behavior of his 16-year-old son, Carlos.

"It was the most unnerving experience. He begged me to take him out for another driving lesson. He can't wait to take his driving test and get his license. I was busy that afternoon, but I made time to do it because I could understand how excited he was about having his first taste of freedom. The lesson went fine and then we come home, and an hour later I was shocked to find him in the basement playing with Legos! I think he would really benefit from therapy."

Mr. Mateo's story provides an example of the normal "madness" that often accompanies adolescence. It was alarming to Mr. Mateo to see how quickly Carlos lunged forward into his impending adulthood, only to retreat an hour later into the world of his childhood. Mr. Mateo's response to his son's developmentally appropriate "madness" was not unusual. He believed Carlos needed help for his strange and contradictory behavior. Mr. Mateo, like many parents we see in therapy, worried that his son's insistence on playing with legos was a clear indication that he did not possess the maturity necessary for driving a car. He was convinced that he had all the information he needed to substantiate his belief that Carlos was a little immature and was probably better served by continuing to play with games at home than to be pushed into the adult world of driving prematurely. Obviously, Carlos disagreed! Furthermore, the different perceptions between him and his dad regarding this matter became a major source of tension, animosity, and conflict in their relationship.

In cases like these, it has been our experience that the adolescent axioms can be helpful as a guide to both professionals and parents. Axiom, for example, serves as a reminder to Mr. Mateo that the period of adolescence can often be considered a state of temporary and developmentally sanctioned insanity. It is helpful for parents, especially those experiencing an adolescent for the first time, to know that the vacillation between extreme behaviors is "normal madness" and not necessarily indicative of anything profoundly or uniquely dysfunctional. In taking such a stance, it becomes a little easier for parents like Mr. Mateo to keep in mind that their appraisal of the adolescent's immaturity may be a little exaggerated, as is the adolescent's appraisal of his or her maturity. For professionals, it can often help us to avoid the trap of colluding with parents about how "bad or mad they are" when we remind and empower ourselves to remind and empower parents to put the behavior into a developmental context. We are not suggesting that seeing the behavior in its developmental context will magically make it less annoying, repulsive, and/or objectionable to a parent. However, we do believe and have certainly found in our work that when parents can accomplish this feat (with lots of support from us) it changes how the parents respond, which ultimately helps to change nonproductive interactions.

Adolescents with acting-out, obnoxious, and rebellious behaviors are also lightning rods for most adults interacting with them. These behaviors are often associated with either kids who have gone bad or those who are a bit worrisome because their behavior flirts with crossing the lines of moral decency and respect. More often than not, parents, teachers, and other professionals working with adolescents are usually concerned with what is often believed to be the clear indicators of "badness." Unfortunately, too many of us typically respond to the "signs" of the once good kids gone or threatening to go bad with increased coercion and control. For example, we routinely hear parents in therapy give their teens some variation of the message "It's *my* way or the *highway*." Ultimatums like this create a "lose–lose" situation for everyone. Many adolescents often feel forced to comply, lie, or say "bye." In each of these cases, adult–adolescent relationships are strained, if not ruptured, over issues that more often than not are developmentally appropriate.

As we indicated earlier, there were times when we responded to the apparent "madness and badness" of teens by trying to either cure or control them. We gradually recognized that we had been assuming their behavior was somehow abnormal or problematic. We had our fantasies about "the good teen" eagerly waiting for us to bestow our wisdom, insight, and guidance on him or her. We were trying to find that adolescent who would see us as benevolent, caring adults and not merely as agents of social control or symbols of the establishment that threatened his or her freedom. In a sense, we were looking for "an easy ride." We were looking for the type of teen who would make things easy for us. We now know that there are "no easy rides," especially in the therapy room.

Embracing the "expect madness, badness, and no easy rides" axiom has been extremely helpful to us. It acknowledges the inevitable struggle and strife that most adolescents experience, and more importantly it reminds us of this during times we most often need a gentle reminder. This axiom normalizes the testing of limits that tends to occur during this stage of development. There is a type of peace that flows from accepting that the mantra many adolescents live by is to "make life miserable for adults." Adults who embrace this reality tend to avoid making the unalterable decisions, ultimatums, and edicts that often result in no-win positions with adolescents.

One of the main advantages we have found to using this axiom as a guiding principle is that it has afforded many families small pieces of hope in the midst of situations that appeared hopeless. When parents are able to see badness and madness as normal within a developmental framework, it makes the task of coping and managing easier. It helps to know that this or that disturbing behavior is part of a phase of development rather than an indictment of one's efficacy as a parent or, worse, the early signs of a malignant psychological condition. As family therapists, we often remind parents that "adolescence is like a bad virus for which there are no antibiotics—it simply has to run its course." Accordingly, we believe it is unfortunate when otherwise healthy and meaningful parent–child relationships get strained during the adolescent stage and never seem to recover because of a failure to effectively negotiate the madness, badness, no easy rides axiom. Our clinical practices are inundated with 35-, 45-, and 50-year-old adults with unfulfilling relationships with parents, and most of these are the ultimate outcome of experiences that went sour during adolescence.

2. Invoke the PTA Rule

The PTA rule asserts that parents, teachers, therapists, and other adults must be "stronger" and "healthier" than the adolescents with whom they interact. PTA refers to parents, teachers, and adults. We use the terms "stronger" and "healthier" in a very specific way. Our definition of strength goes beyond the traditional notion of brute force. Instead, we think of strength as an emotional attribute that stems from having the capacity to appropriately manage one's own emotions and another's simultaneously. This "emotional skill" requires emotional health, which stems from having a sense of inner security and psychological wholeness. Maddy and her 15-year-old daughter, Sheila, were engaged in the classic parent–adolescent power struggle over rules and boundaries. During our third therapy session, Sheila told her mother that she wanted the freedom to go out Saturday night and permission to come home at 1:00 AM. Maddy refused. She said she needed to think about whether or not Sheila could go out at all, but—either way—she would not be allowed to stay out past 10:00 P.M. Sheila was livid.

"I hate you," Sheila screamed. "You're trying to ruin my life. All you want to do is control me. I hate you! I hate you and I wish you weren't my mother!" The air in our small therapy room was thick with the emotional intensity that was raging between Sheila and her mother.

"You hate me? Well, guess what—I hate you too! You think I like having to waste my time with this bullshit conflict? Don't you think I have better things to do with my time than worry about who you're running around with and what trouble you're trying to get into? I really regret the day I had labor pains to have you!"

Given Sheila's attacking and hurtful words, Maddy's response to her daughter was understandable. However, we have found that it is not terribly helpful to engage in an escalating game of "tit for tat" with adolescents. While it probably felt good at the moment to snap back at her daughter with equal venom and hostility, in the end Maddy's response did little to help the situation. Instead, we believe it would have been more effective for Maddy to invoke the PTA rule. In so doing, we believe she would have been better able to see Sheila's outburst for what it was: a tantrum from a frustrated young person who felt trapped and powerless and who was raging against the one person who seemed to be blocking her pathway to freedom. Admittedly, although not easy to do, the situation required Maddy to see beyond the "grenade-slinging outbursts" of Sheila and respond to her in a loving and reassuring way. To one-up her daughter with an anger-laced grenade-slinging outburst of her own did very little to bring mother and daughter closer. For a variety of reasons Maddy was unable to respond to Sheila, at least on this occasion, in a way that was productive and facilitative.

There are as many varied reasons for why it may be difficult for some parents to invoke the PTA rule, particularly when it is most needed. These reasons range from stress to poor parenting skills to varying philosophies regarding parent–child interactions. While we possess neither the space nor the knowledge to account for all the potential impediments there are to executing the PTA axiom, we would like to discuss one of the most common factors underpinning the difficulty that parents and other adults sometimes have in invoking the PTA rule.

Relational Contaminants: Unresolved Conflicts, Thoughts, and Feelings

Adolescents by the very nature of who they are have a unique ability to activate old (unresolved) conflicts, worries, or feelings that some adults have left over from their adolescence or earlier family experiences. When old thoughts, feelings, and conflicts (re)emerge in our contemporary interactions, they have a way of contaminating communications. In our therapy, we refer to the reemergence of these leftover issues, particularly those that block functional interactions, as relational contaminants. We think of them as contaminants because of the negative effects that they tend to have on relationships. The presence of relational contaminants makes it difficult for interactions in the here and now to remain in the present.

When adults like Maddy have difficulty in invoking the PTA rule, such difficulties often are rooted in unresolved issues from the past that involve unfulfilled needs and/or expectations, or relational contaminants. Ironically, it is not uncommon to note that relational contaminants can be unexpectedly activated in the midst of our daily efforts to live life under the most mundane circumstances. It does not take a major societal event or a key family event to set off a relational contaminant; it can and often happens benignly.

Over the years we have found that adolescents, in particular, seem to be lightning rods for many of the unresolved issues that adults harbor within themselves. Hence, when adults come into contact with teens, they tend to be quite vulnerable to having their relational contaminants triggered during these interactions. When this occurs, adults suddenly find that they are no longer dealing with whatever the issue of the moment is but instead are caught up in feelings and sensations tied to the past. The triggering of unresolved issues from the past brings forth a flood of memories and emotions that makes it exceedingly difficult to invoke the PTA rule. We have identified two common sources of relational contaminants that commonly prevent healthy constructive adult–adolescent interactions, namely: family of origin; and peers and partners.

Family of Origin. Adults who have unresolved issues rooted in their family of origin can struggle with unfulfilled needs and expectations with respect to parents, siblings, grandparents, and/or any other relative. For example, in Maddy's case, she could not be "stronger and healthier" than Sheila because of relational contamination involving her relationship with her own mother. Maddy had struggled her entire life with not feeling wanted or loved by her own mother. When she was 5, her mother had told her she never wanted her, that she was "an accident." It was a devastating thing for a parent to say to a child. Maddy openly admitted that her mother's disclosure had scarred her deeply.

When Maddy was 18, she married her high school sweetheart, and a year later Sheila was born. The marriage fell apart when Sheila was 4 months old, and Maddy became and remained a single mother. She was hurt and disappointed about the failure of her marriage but grateful that she had Sheila. She vowed to give her daughter all the love she felt she had been deprived of as a child.

> "It's always been hard for me to support both of us with no one else to help, but I always thought it was worth it because of the love between me and Sheila. Now, all of that has changed. She's moody and selfish. All she thinks about now is wanting to go out with her friends. She is really selfish."

Maddy's need to derive love and affirmation from her relationship with Sheila impaired her ability to tolerate the natural stresses and strains of Sheila's adolescence. Maddy interpreted Sheila's normal inclinations toward individuation and autonomy as signs of rejection. Maddy responded to her hurt and insecurity by trying to control Sheila more strictly, which eventually led to the eruption in therapy. Maddy's painful experiences with rejection made it exceedingly difficult for her to be stronger and healthier than Sheila. Instead of dealing effectively with both Sheila's feelings and her own, she was consumed by her own pain and suffering. She lashed back at Sheila, which had the effect of creating further distance between them.

Peers and Partners. "Peers" refers to friends as well as acquaintances who usually, although not necessarily always, share membership in a common cohort group. Partners are those with whom one shares an intimate romantic relationship. Relational contaminants that stem from relationships with peers or partners involve unfulfilled needs and expectations related to one's friends, acquaintances, or romantic partners.

Mr. Laven, a 10th-grade teacher in an inner-city high school, blew a fuse when Ricky, a student in his class, criticized his Hunter green golf shirt. In classic adolescent-like fashion, Ricky's timing was impeccable. He and a group of his friends were in the gymnasium when Mr. Laven entered with three female colleagues. Ricky, after skillfully gaining everyone's attention, began to make a series of wisecracks about the shirt. His cracks generated raucous laughter that echoed throughout the gymnasium. Mr. Laven's face turned beet-red.

"You think you're funny, don't you, Ricky? Well, look at whose talking? You'll probably have to repeat 10th-grade English again. You can barely string together two grammatically correct sentences. The one thing around here that seems laughable is the thought that you might ever graduate from this school and make something of your life."

Ricky's smile vanished. The sound of laughter was quickly transformed into a tomb of silence. It was obvious to everyone looking on that Ricky was deeply wounded by the comment. Mr. Laven now looked smug and content.

Suddenly Ricky's eyes squinted, and he stepped forward, saying: "Hey, fuck you, man, with your rich-boy preppy attitude!"

Mr. Laven was enraged all over again. "What did you say, you little punk? Who the hell do you think you're talking to like that—your father? Oh, yeah, you probably don't have a father. That must be your problem. Get down to the office now!"

This interaction quickly escalated into a bitter conflict that spiraled out of control. Because Mr. Laven failed to invoke the PTA rule, what started out as a teenager trying to tease an adult quickly degenerated into a much more vicious encounter that resulted in a 2-day suspension for Ricky.

It would have been helpful for Mr. Laven to understand the deeper motive behind Ricky's behavior. Perhaps Ricky's comments were purely benign, intended in as spirit of good fun. Or maybe he really wanted to hurt and humiliate his teacher. Even if the latter were the case, why did Ricky need to do this? Was he angry with Mr. Laven for something? Had his teacher hurt or offended him in some way? If so, it would be much more helpful to deal with these issues rather than getting into an increasingly nasty game of verbal one-upmanship.

Because Mr. Laven wasn't able to check his own emotions long enough to try to understand the emotional roots of Ricky's wise-cracks, he missed an opportunity to deescalate the situation and repair whatever strains obviously existed in his relationship with Ricky.

In fairness to Mr. Laven, it is much easier to discuss the PTA rule as an abstract concept than it is to execute it in the midst of difficult human interactions. When we explained our position to Mr. Laven, he replied that he had handled the situation with strength: he met Ricky head on and showed him that "I'm not going to take his crap." Obviously, our definition of strength differed from Mr. Laven's. To him, strength involved demonstrating to Ricky that he could beat him at his own game. For us, strength resided in Mr. Laven's ability to endure Ricky's criticism long enough to get to whatever was at the root of the behavior. Our notion of strength would have been for Mr. Laven to have accomplished this task without lashing back in a vengeful and retaliatory fashion.

Upon closer examination, what we discovered was that when Mr. Laven was an adolescent he suffered greatly with the pain of social isolation and rejection from his peers. He felt utterly alone, unable to fit in with any of the kids his age. He spent most of his time alone reading or building model planes. Far from developing a positive sense of identity, his sense of himself was that of a social misfit—an outcast. Following completion of high school Mr. Laven attended college. Because he was a good student he succeeded academically, but his social and emotional distance from peers persisted. Eventually he earned his masters degree, and shortly thereafter he began teaching math at the same high school where he still teaches today. Outwardly Mr. Laven seemed to have developed a successful life in spite of the awkwardness and pain of his adolescence.

Although he had a reputation as a stern—sometimes too stern—disciplinarian, Mr. Laven also was well known for his high standards and academic excellence. It was easy enough to recognize that, underneath it all, Mr. Laven was still the emotionally insecure, easily hurt, socially awkward young teenager who felt rejected by his peers. The only difference was that in his role as an adult and teacher he had access to power that allowed him to hide his vulnerabilities in a way he could not as a youth. He now had ways of protecting himself that were not available to him 20 years earlier.

Whenever Mr. Laven was faced with a teenager like Ricky who triggered such painful memories from his past, he found himself reliving the humiliation and rejection from peers that had wounded him during his adolescence. All of his excruciating insecurities came flooding back, and his instinctive reaction to pull away and protect himself was overwhelming. He was incapable of reflecting upon what might be going on for someone like Ricky, because in those moments he wasn't relating from the perspective of an adult but rather that of an adolescent. As such, Mr. Laven could not fathom containing his feelings long enough to respond appropriately to Ricky's baiting comment. He was too overwhelmed by his own emotions. This is a classic example of how relational contaminants related to past peer relationships can interfere with effectively invoking the PTA rule.

In the next chapter we will provide a specific tool that can be used to facilitate invoking the PTA rule during volatile situations. We believe that utilizing the PTA rule enables those of us interacting with adolescents to refrain from sliding down the same slippery slope that so many teens are sliding down when they feel frustrated, hopeless, disrespected, and increasingly out of control.

Whether tied to experiences with one's family of origin, peers, partners, or some other significant other, we believe it is important to identify and find ways to address one's relational contaminants. We believe this is particularly vital to do since there is a very strong connection between the presence of relational contaminants and the degrees of difficulty experienced in invoking the PTA rule effectively.

When adults are able to invoke the PTA rule, they can respond like Ellen, a mother of three, when her 14-year-old son Robby screamed: "I hate your guts! You're nothing but a loser!" Appearing momentarily unbalanced, Ellen took a deep breath and then answered: "Well, I can understand how you feel. There were times when I was 14 that I hated my parents too. I just want you to know that I still love you."

Ellen's response to Robby was a good example of how to invoke the PTA rule. Invoking the PTA rule means that the adult recognizes that it is his or her responsibility to find the strength, courage, and patience to respond in ways that deescalate conflict. Put-downs, especially by those in authority, often incite rather than reduce conflict. While an adult might derive momentary catharsis from counterattacking, whether by direct hostile engagement or by passive (punitive) withdrawal from the interaction, this does little to strengthen an already stressed relationship.

Challenges Faced by Therapists and Other Professionals Invoking the PTA Rule

For therapists and other professionals working with adolescents, invoking the PTA rule can also be challenging for a variety of reasons. First, as professionals, we are certainly susceptible to the same relational contaminant difficulties and blindspots that plague those we treat in therapy. Unfortunately, much of our work often occurs in a context where what we say is not always subject to close scrutiny. Hence, our inappropriate or ill-advised comments or responses to adolescents may either remain undetected or be dismissed or catalogued as a professionally grounded response based on clinical expertise. The case of Mrs. Moody provides a good example of the point we are suggesting here.

Mrs. Moody was a counselor in a residential treatment center for "emotionally disturbed" and "adjudicated youth." She had been employed for 18 years at the same facility and was very well respected by her colleagues as well as by many of the youth in her unit. During one of our consultation visits to the facility, we had the opportunity to observe Mrs. Moody in the midst of an acrimonious exchange with 13-year-old Tawanna.

"I'm gonna ask you one time and one time only, Tawanna, to get the hell out of my sight! I can't stand to look at you for even a second, I am so pissed and disgusted with you . . Leave now before I mess around and get locked up for doing something I might regret," Mrs. Moody angrily said to Tawanna. She had just discovered that the teen was 4 months pregnant. Tawanna seemed stunned by Mrs. Moody's enraged response. She stood frozen, seemingly unable to flex a single muscle, with tears quickly forming and streaming down her face. She seemed hurt and embarrassed. Mrs. Moody, on the other hand, seemed unfazed by Tawanna's obvious signs of devastation and emotional unraveling. In a harsh and scolding voice, she continued to repeat: "LEAVE! "I SAID, LEAVE!"

This was a painfully difficult interaction to observe. When we discussed the interaction with others in the facility, we were amazed by the feedback we received. Mrs. Moody's colleagues expressed a range of reactions not just to the Tawanna interaction but to her style in general. There were many who considered her to be a little too harsh and at times abusive with the kids; however, none of them had ever discussed this with her. Many of her colleagues stated some variation of the following theme: "She gets results, and who am I to question or confront her? . . . She has spent most of her life here, and she has an approach that works for her and the kids . . . These are the lessons you learn after working in a place like this for as long as she has."

When we spoke to Mrs. Moody, she admitted that she "had lost it a little bit." She explained she loved Tawanna as she would a daughter and that she had "preached to her a million times about not getting caught up in the teen pregnancy trap," a life she herself had learned about the hard way, as a single-parent teenaged mother. In retrospect, Mrs. Moody believed that her love and concern for Tawanna's well-being justified her reaction. As she stated to us repeatedly, "I have been doing this work for 18 years, and you don't stay at a place like this for this long by kissing up to these kids . . . They only respond to toughness . . . If they sense you are weak, they take advantage of you."

We highlight this vignette regarding Mrs. Moody, her colleagues, and Tawanna for several reasons. We believe it again puts a spotlight on how difficult it is to implement the PTA rule and that this is true for professionals as well as nonprofessionals. We believe it underscores some of the inherent challenges that those of us who work with adolescents must face not only in executing the PTA but also in detecting our failure to do so. Mrs. Moody's professional stature and years of service, made it virtually impossible for her and those with whom she worked to consider that perhaps there was a better way in which she could communicate with the adolescents. She was revered and extolled among her peers for "the respect she demanded from the kids." Yet, the *respect* that they often spoke of, to our outsiders' eyes, too often seemed like fear.

We had numerous opportunities to observe Mrs. Moody's work, and we were consistently impressed with her dedication to "my kids," as she referred to them. She had excellent rapport with most of the adolescents in the facility, which was no small feat. Yet, in spite of all the ways in which she worked well with the youth, she, perhaps like all of us, had some rather serious blindspots that seemed to interfere with her ability to be more nurturing and emotionally available to the likes of Tawanna. This, to us, was unfortunate, since the desire for nurturance and having someone there for them was an insatiable hunger that most of her "kids" craved.

Attempting to invoke the PTA rule in therapy sessions can also be challenging at times. Family therapy is particularly a challenge in this regard, because it is not uncommon to have multiple participants in the consulting room, all with competing needs and agendas. We have experienced on more than one occasion that when adolescents in therapy say things to us that seem belligerent or inappropriate, parents frequently are irritated when we do not respond in a punitive manner. At times, each of us has received lashings from parents that rival the lashings we received from their adolescents. In these instances, we usually learn firsthand what it's like to be an adolescent in these particular families. The criticisms we have received on these occasions all point toward the same theme: "we should fight fire with fire." Unfortunately, we know this strategy is doomed to failure. For all the fortitude and might it requires to respond nonreactively while being verbally assaulted, we are quick to remind parents that we've already tried getting tough with teens who were tough with us. It never helped.

It's only through accumulated experiences that we have learned the wisdom of invoking the PTA axiom. It has been infinitely more helpful to disarm verbal bombers with empathy and validation. When Molina, a 16-year-old girl, shouted in therapy that we (referring to her parents as well as the two of us as her therapists) could all "go burn in hell!" it was tempting to lash back at her. Instant rage registered on the faces of her parents, who clearly wanted to counterattack. Her parents were obviously insulted and embarrassed. Before they could respond verbally, we said to Molina: "You seem really angry with all of us right now, which if you are is quite understandable." Shocked by this seemingly "soft reply," Molina's father bellowed: "What do you think you're doing? You're condoning my daughter's filthy mouth and her miserable attitude. This is not what I brought her to therapy for. If you can't deal with an out-of-control adolescent, we'll find someone who can."

Our response to Molina was disappointing to her father. He wanted, and certainly thought that her outburst warranted, a more assertive response from us. Our failure to provide it triggered an ultimatum from him and the threat to fire us as his family's therapists. In situations like these, which are fairly common in treatment, we have found that a PTA-type response from us to the father is most helpful. We have found it useful to avoid critical, confrontational responses to parents even when they have been critical and confrontational with us. This stance is predicated on our firm belief in the PTA rule. In other words, not only do we believe that parents and adults have a responsibility to promote and maintain *healthy* interactions with young people rather than strained and destructive ones; but also assume that therapists and other professionals should ensure that we maintain meaningful, productive relationships even with frustrated, irate parents who challenge our clinical judgment and expertise.

While our experiences with adolescents have confirmed the benefits of invoking the PTA rule, we try to remain ever mindful of the ways that inner hurts, insecurities, and fears can make it difficult to invoke this rule. Adults with unresolved issues from their own past, especially their adolescence, sometimes struggle to access the inner strength and health that are needed to disarm a verbal bomber through validation and compassion. For this reason, a salient aspect of our work with adults who interact with adolescents involves encouraging them to do their emotional homework. It is important for all of us, as adults, to heal the hurts that haunt us so that we can be strong and healthy enough to "rise above" the errant verbal missiles that teens so often send our way.

3. Be Suspicious of Memory

This axiom is predicated on the notion that so many of us often rely heavily on the memories of our glorified past as a reference point for working with and understanding today's adolescents. We cannot count the number of times that we have heard form parents and professionals about "the way we were." And it is usually not just the way we were but how the way we were was so much better. "We were never as disrespectful as today's kids . . . We had things we feared . . . cared about . . . In my day we had more self-respect than to walk around with our underwear showing—and the girls are as bad as the boys are today—it wasn't that way when I was a kid" and so on. These are the types of assessments that we make of today's adolescents based on our memories about the glorified past. Our memories, reflections, and comparisons usually leave many of us concluding that today's youth are among the worst ever. Because they are bad kids who are among the worst ever, we believe we need more control, more children criminally tried as adults, more prisons, more detention centers, more sedative drugs, and ultimately more punishment and restraints.

While we would be the first to argue that it is crucial for us to remember that we too were once adolescents, we think it is also prudent to be a little suspicious of our memories. A common trap that many adults working with adolescents slip into is to use the memories of their adolescence as a reference point for judging and evaluating the experiences of today's youth. There is little that is problematic about these types of memories, especially if we are also "suspicious" of the purity of our recall. We have found that memories of the glorious days become problematic when they become fixed unscrutinized points of reference. When this happens adolescents get locked into a set of expectations based largely on fantasy. The danger this poses lies in the selective nature of memory. Especially as we grow older, memory is prone to becoming increasingly *kind and generous* to many of us. Each of us has had experiences in our respective lives that have been slightly rewritten, perhaps a little embellished over the course of time. We remember some small seemingly insignificant detail as we had hoped it was rather than as it really was—for example, the dance recital that was executed to perfection when we recall it decades later, or the pure raw talent that was consistently displayed during a distinguished little league career that probably has far more luster now than it did three decades ago.

I (TAL) had an experience that underscored the highly subjective character of memory. A number of years ago, my sister and I, who are 2 years apart in age, were talking casually. At that time we were each in our early 20s. My sister, Joyce, mentioned that we seemed to be so much less competitive with each other now than we were growing up. I was stunned by her comment because, as I could recall, I had never been competitive with her. While I believed she had always felt competitive with me, I was convinced it was a one-way competition.

"No offense, Sis," I said with amusement, "but I've never felt competitive with you. I remember times when I know you tried to compete with me, but I never bought into that with you. I just never felt that way toward you. I was too concerned about trying to be supportive of you."

With a tinge of irritation Joyce responded by saying, "I'll admit I competed with you, but you competed with me too. I'm not saying that was bad—it was a sister thing—but please don't try to tell me now that you were this little angel."

"I know I wasn't angelic, but neither was I competitive with you. The fact is: to compete, I would have had to believe you had something I wanted, or that you were going to get something I wanted. I'm telling you: I never felt that with you. I am positive about this."

Needless to say, Joyce was annoyed by my assertion that I never competed with her. I certainly did not want to insult her, but I was absolutely convinced that I was right. To this day I would still be convinced that my memory of our childhood together was serving me accurately had I not found a journal entry I had written when I was 11. The entry read as follows:

"Every time my sister and I are talking to someone or being introduced, the same thing happens. Everyone calls me "the dancer," but when they talk about Joyce, they say everything from she's going to be a political genius (President is what they mean to say), to she's an electronics wizard, she a meticulous house cleaner, a talented entertainer, a fantastic writer, a stupendous cook, a brilliant photographer, and even a great tractor driver. Is there anything she isn't good at? What should I do? It's not that I'm against Joyce. But what about me? How many times have I been dancing and then I'm rudely interrupted by my talented, entertaining sister who takes over the whole show. Everyone thinks she is so great—and she is great—but why does she always have to be the center of everyone's attention? And then, of course, not to mention how many times have I worked on a project for months and then suddenly along she comes and suddenly starts the same project. Of course, she only works on hers a few days, but everyone raves about her."

I was horrified when I read this journal entry, because it revealed a part of my past that I had completely forgotten or repressed. Had I not read my words written in my own hand, I would never have believed it. I still find it difficult to accept that I wrote those words or, more to the point, that I had these feelings. But there it was—my intense competition with my sister, which my memory as an adult had conveniently selected out. I had no recollection of any of the stories or feelings mentioned in my journal until I stumbled across it a dozen years later. It demonstrated for me beyond a doubt just how suspect memory truly is!

While memory, and its susceptibility to innocent distortion, is essentially harmless, it can be potentially inflammatory when used as a barometer for judging adolescents. Whether conscious or not, intentional or unintentional, it is common for adults to use their adolescence as a reference point for making all types of judgments about today's adolescents. We believe this is not only difficult but dangerous as well. When we fail to critically examine and reflect upon our adolescent-age experiences, we can unwittingly set standards and have expectations that are unrealistic for many youth today. It may very well be that "kids today are more disrespectful and violent" than were their counterparts of any other generation, and it is equally possible that times have changed so dramatically that it is difficult to judge today's youth by yesterday's mores, values, and standards. Having taken this position, we are not suggesting that the wisdom and knowledge we gained from our adolescence is worthless. Instead, we are suggesting that is useful for each of us to simultaneously remember that we were once adolescents and that our respective *memories are suspect* and should be scrutinized. When this feat is accomplished, we are all reminded, as Mike and the Mechanics sang in "Living Years," that "every generation blames the one before."

We use the "be suspicious of memory" axiom in therapy in several useful ways. As a matter of common clinical practice with adolescents and their families, we routinely ask parents to reflect on their childhood and adolescence. Then we invite them to examine and discuss how their attitudes, beliefs, and behaviors were regarded by their parents and other adults. This discussion is often followed by inviting their parents, siblings, or other significant family members to the next session. The extended family session is a significant one because among the many therapeutic things that occur are poignant reminders of why we should be suspicious of memory. Invariably during this session, there are recurring debates about the details of a memory— either varying recollections or interpretations. This process provides a much needed foundation for a series of conversations that we have with parents about the purity of the memories that they rely upon in parenting their adolescent. We believe that when memories are scrutinized they can be used to liberate interactions with adolescents, and when they are not they tend to promote a kind of interpersonal incarceration. Scrutinizing the memory of one's adolescent years allows parents to focus on the process issues associated with the developmental period such as the importance of peer acceptance, changes in one's body, and so on. When memories remain pure, there is a tendency to innocently exaggerate the way it used to be.

4. Differentiate between Style and Substance

It probably wasn't some breathtaking, pivotal moment in therapy that led to our undying and unwavering commitment to this axiom. Instead, it was probably something altogether more personal. For example, in my (KVH) case, I believe it was probably the unrelenting, highly alarmed voice of Clarence Hardy, my father, that highlighted the salience of this axiom for me. Undoubtedly, it didn't really happen in the way I am about to report (since memory is suspect), but this is how I remember it some three decades later.

During my adolescence, Afros, which required long, untreated hair, were an integral part of the uniform of my generation. Peers issued merit points for "the brother or sister" who had the longest, best-shaped, and best-groomed "fro," as they were commonly called. The merit points issued by admiring, attractive girls made wearing the fro even more appealing—at least it did for me. I wore a fro that was both a source of attention and distraction. But, as anyone from that generation knows, what good was a decent fro without all of the other aesthetic generational trappings? So, in the spirit of my generational norms, my fro was often accompanied by at least 20 silver snake-headed bangles on my wrist and a 4-inch-wide silver medallion of a scorpion (my Zodiac sign) attached to a leather rawhide cord that hung around my neck. I wore multicolored, flared bell-bottom jeans bearing the names of my girlfriend, peers, and statements reflecting my political views on issues ranging from capital punishment to the War on Poverty. By my standards, my carefully groomed and well-orchestrated presentation to the world affirmed what my peers frequently proclaimed: "Kenny's cool."

However, to my father my carefully cultivated look was a warning sign that his lovable, decent son was on a perilous downward spiral to nowhere. "I never thought I would see the day when a son of mine would have more hair than his mother!" he once exclaimed in a state of utter disbelief.

Although some aspect of my generational uniform seemed to earn the scorn of parents, teachers, and clergy, it never once deterred my inclination or my ability to do well academically. Sure, it took me an extra 20–30 minutes in the morning to get the fro perfectly symmetrical, but I never missed school. Whatever sleep I lost by having to get up a little earlier to get it all together was a small price to pay for the rewards bestowed upon me by admiring peers. For me, it was a no-brainer! Yes, it did make wearing a baseball cap nearly impossible, but it didn't prevent me from being an avid baseball fan and player. The errors I made on the field were unrelated to the length of my hair or how high I wore my socks.

Sometimes I think we forget that every generation has a uniform, a style of dress, a way of speaking, and an approach to hair that are markers of an era. And although these uniforms may be outrageous, disgusting, and embarrassing to adults, for many adolescents they constitute a source of pride, a declaration of one's membership in a given generation. Thus, our axiom is that it is best to appoint adolescents as the superintendents of style and have parents worry about the substantive issues. Whether a child goes to school is a matter of substance, while the decision to wear a belt is a style issue. Whether an adolescent does drugs, drinks and drives, or glorifies violence are all salient substantive issues. Wearing Dad's boxers to the mall—although troubling for many parents who relate to them only as underwear—doesn't qualify in our book as a substantive issue in isolation.

In our work it has been helpful for us to continually draw critical distinctions between style and substance. Doing so has enabled us to refrain from the inevitable mistake of imposing myriad stylistically based preconditions that adolescents have to meet in order for therapy to occur. "Please sit down" . . . "don't swivel in the chair" . . . "Take off the sunglasses" (and on and on) are all nonsubstantive issues that could create a gulf between the therapist and the adolescent in therapy—but only if you let them. Even before our caseloads began to shift toward working with more aggressive adolescents, we began to realize that having the opportunity to impact young people didn't require us to be the experts on style. Whether one sits or stands in therapy seems to have absolutely no effect on the outcome of therapy! How we respond to it, on the other hand, does.

In the best of circumstances, distinguishing between style and substance would be simple, clean, and clear-cut with no shades of gray. Unfortunately, there are always some cases in which the distinction between style and substance is somewhat murky. For instance, we continue to struggle around the process of body piercing and tattoos. Our work with violent adolescents has made this an even more critical, much harder, call. There are approaches to piercing (and tattooing) that suggest it is a necessary accessory to the uniform of today's generation. On the other hand, there are versions of the very same behavior that seem less style-oriented and much more diagnostic of serious substantive issues (Selekman & O'Hanlon, 2002). The extent to and conditions under which adolescents engage in piercing, along with the motivations that underpin it, must be carefully examined within the context of this axiom to distinguish between style and substance.

In clinical settings and with families alike, this axiom provides all of us who interact closely with adolescents with a framework to help us better pick the struggles that we believe are worthy of haggling over. In therapy we typically surrender the issues of style to the adolescent, and we strongly urge parents to do the same. On the other hand, we are far more likely to "dig in" where the "life-and-death" substantive issues are concerned.

5. Recognize How Adolescents Are Similar Yet Different

While adolescents share much in common, they also have many differences between and among them. For example, all adolescents are faced with the same developmental tasks (i.e., establishing an identity and finding a way to achieve a healthy balance between the forces of separation and connection), but each young person finds unique ways of negotiating these tasks. Although Keanna, age 17, and Taniqua, age 15, are sisters, their parents, Benita and James Jordan, were amazed by how different their daughters are from each other.

"We raised them in the same family, but they turned out so different," said James.

"Keanna has always been extremely responsible, maybe over-responsible," Benita explained. "She always loved school and always got straight A's. She couldn't care less about socializing with friends. She's wanted to be a doctor since she was 6 and has read about every book in the library. She is very family-oriented. She spends a lot of time around here helping with my mother, who's quite old and needs a lot of care. Taniqua, on the other hand, is totally the opposite. She doesn't know what she wants to do with her life. First she wanted to be a dancer, then a singer, photographer, gymnast, writer, and now she's thinking maybe she'll just move to New York City when she graduates from high school and will explore different things. She's always been eager to go out and explore the world. She can't wait to leave, and Keanna would be content never leaving. In fact, Keanna's enrolling at a college in the area and living at home."

The Jordans' descriptions of their daughters reveal how both Keanna and Taniqua are dealing with similar developmental tasks. Each is striving to seek out, define, and assert her unique identity, and each is wrestling with how to balance the competing forces of separation and connection. Yet, the pathways each has chosen are quite different. Keanna has a clear vision of her future and what she wants to do with her life. She also is extremely connected with her family. What is less clear is how she will find a way to retain her strong family ties while also taking steps toward greater independence and autonomy.

Taniqua's search for her identity seems less focused and clear than Keanna's. She is searching to find her niche in the world; however, she seems very open to the process of exploration. Unlike her sister, Taniqua seems much more comfortable with not having everything laid out in front of her. Moreover, she seems eager to fly away from "the nest" and establish her autonomy. In Taniqua's case, there is little doubt that she is capable of separating from her family. However, only time will tell how she will manage to forge her independence while also retaining a meaningful connection with her family. The Jordan sisters wonderfully illustrate the importance of recognizing how adolescents are both similar and different. For example, Keanna was born into a family where there were no other children present to inexperienced, highly anxious first-time parents. Her sister, on the other hand, was born into a family where from birth she had a sibling as well as parents who were a little more experienced. We believe these small, subtle differences are huge and often account for the otherwise unexplainable differences that exist among siblings.

To some, this point may seem obvious, but we have heard numerous perplexed parents who have said things like "Why did this child turned out so differently from the others. They all grew up in the same family . . . We loved them all the same, so why did this one go astray?" The point that is often overlooked in situations like these is that no two children grow up in precisely the same family. The simple fact of one's birth order may create vastly different experiences of one's family.

Adolescents also share certain features in common that make them distinctly recognizable as a group. For instance, they tend to share a common language, codes of dress, mores, and values. In a sense, adolescents have their own culture. And yet, despite their shared membership in the culture of adolescence, significant variations and diversity exist among members of this group. These differences are shaped by "informants" that may include—although they are not necessarily limited to—race, class, gender, sexual orientation, religion, regionality, ethnicity, family constellation, and exposure to and experiences with technology. We use the term "informants" because we believe these factors "inform" how adolescents interpret, negotiate, and work toward the resolution of a host of developmentally appropriate tasks.

Tiffany Wellington and Mi Ling Young are both 17. They attend the same high school and have been friends for 3 years. They wear each other's clothes, exchange CDs of their favorite musical artists, and communicate in a "language" that is completely foreign to their parents and teachers. However, Tiffany and Mi Ling are by no means carbon copies. Tiffany's family traces its history in the United States back to the *Mayflower*. Her ancestors grew to enjoy the benefits of great wealth, but the family fortune was lost during the stock market crash of 1929. Since that time her family has struggled economically. Mi Ling's family immigrated to the United States from Taiwan when she was 7 years old. Her family is financially successful and has never had to worry about money.

Both families want their daughters to establish a secure future for themselves in terms of money and marriage. Tiffany is the youngest child, with two older brothers. Her parents saved for years to send her oldest brother to college, and her younger brother enlisted in the army. Her parents' hope for her is that she will marry a financially successful man thereby establishing an economically secure base for herself. Tiffany finds this insulting. Although she is a heterosexual and wants to marry a man one day, she objects to her parents' notion that the only way for her to succeed in life is by marrying a wealthy man. "I understand my parents' concerns about money. I don't want to live by just getting by for the rest of my life, but I don't want to have to get hitched right after high school and become a housewife just for the bank account." Instead, Tiffany wants to move to Hollywood after high school and try to make it as an actress. She has been very direct with her parents about her plans in spite of their protestations.

As an only child, Mi Ling's parents have invested all their hope and dreams in her. They expect that she will attend college to become a doctor. They also expect that she will meet and marry a man of comparable educational and career status. Mi Ling shares her parents' career goals for herself. "I have always wanted to be a doctor since I was a little girl. Also, as an Asian American, I have had to face a lot of racism and discrimination, which have inspired me even more to want to work hard and become a success as a doctor." However, she does not know how to tell her parents that she is a lesbian and will never have the heterosexual relationship they want for her. She suffers greatly holding this secret inside, fearful of the reaction her parents would have if she were to tell them the truth about herself.

Despite the bonds of friendship and generation, informants such as race, ethnicity, culture, sexual orientation, class, and family constellation underpin a variety of salient differences between Tiffany and Mi Ling. Therefore, while it is true that all adolescents share a common experience in the sense that they are faced with similar developmental dilemmas and are members of a distinctive cultural group, the lives and experiences of all adolescents are not equal or the same. In our work, we believe it is essential to examine the relationship between these informants and adolescent development and behavior.

CONCLUSION

These adolescent axioms have proven to be enormously helpful to us over the years. Irrespective of the personality of the adolescent or the issues he or she is dealing with, these axioms have provided us with a practical, no-nonsense foundation for our work. They offer a basis for understanding the nature of adolescence in general and for recognizing the typical triggers that "get in our way" and have the potential to undermine our interactions with teens even when violence is not an issue. So many of the clinical strategies we employ with violent and aggressive youth draw heavily on these axioms. They have been a solid foundation upon which our work has rested, yet so much more is needed when working with violent and aggressive youth. In subsequent chapters we will discuss our work with violent youth more specifically.

CHAPTER 7

• • • • • • •

Counteracting Devaluation

Devaluation is a major force shaping the lives of violent adolescents, and it is critical to assume an active role in willfully counteracting it. As stated earlier, devaluation assaults a person's sense of humanity, dignity, and worth. Even situations when the experience that led to devaluation is long over, the emotional effects of the assault, if untreated and unhealed, persist. For those young people who suffer from devaluation, they share in common an underlying emotional injury and a susceptibility to messages that are disparaging, shameful, or rejecting. Consequently, counteracting devaluation in the lives of violent adolescents must consist of providing high doses of affirmation, nurturance, and consideration for the person's dignity and humanity. Both the messages that are sent and the styles of interaction that are utilized must repair and fortify adolescents' sense of themselves. To assist with this objective in this chapter we present several strategies that can be used to counteract devaluation in the lives of violent teens.

THE VCR APPROACH

Unfortunately, many of us unintentionally find ourselves contributing to, rather than counteracting, devaluation in the lives of young people. Whether it's their innocent antics or their insidious antisocial acts, adolescents who act out tend to provoke "C" reactions from adults—challenging, confronting, criticizing, and correcting. While these types of reactions are understandable, they are rarely helpful.

149

Rather than leading to a corrective experience, a barrage of C reactions typically results in adolescents tuning out: they turn a deaf ear. They hear the C reactions as evidence that adults just don't get it. From their perspective, these messages serve as further proof that adults are more concerned with ruling rather than relating, and with lecturing rather than listening. The problem of jumping in too quickly with a C reaction is that it almost always results in perpetuating devaluation. For adolescents, drowning in a sea of devaluation, C reactions intensify their sense of shame and worthlessness, which ultimately undermines the broader objective of redirecting misguided adolescent behavior.

When conducting workshops, we always emphasize the pitfalls of moving too quickly to challenge and criticize adolescents for their wrongdoings. Inevitably, some portion of the audience always has an immediate negative knee-jerk reaction. They explain that they are disturbed to hear us advocating for what, in their minds, is anarchy. As one participant once said to us, "Are you suggesting that when kids do crazy things we should just let them? I think this is terribly irresponsible of you. I know that kids don't like it when we have to be the heavy and lay down the law, but if we don't, then they think they can just keep doing wrong, and then they never learn." This comment is representative of those we receive from many adults with whom we speak. We understand the sentiment and believe that there is considerable validity to the concern. We agree that acting-out adolescents require adult intervention and guidance so they can learn more effective ways of coping with life. Our point is simply that *how* one intervenes is of critical significance. Often the good intentions of adults working with adolescents don't always produce the desired results. In fact, depending upon the vulnerability of the adolescent in question, and the severity of the intervention that is used, it is possible to cause more harm than good.

Through our work with violent and aggressive adolescents, their parents, and other concerned adults, we have developed a strategy for redirecting misguided behaviors and counteracting devaluation. We call this *strategy* the VCR approach. Although we commonly use and refer to the VCR as a technique or strategy, it is purely neither. At one level, the *VCR approach* really represents a worldview, a kind of philosophy about human beings, especially kids who commit horrible acts of violence. When the VCR is considered much more broadly than a technique or strategy, it asserts the position that all human beings— even bad kids—possess redeemable qualities that are of value. We believe that embracing this perspective enables us to fully appreciate that bad kids can commit good deeds and that good kids on occasion do in fact commit misdeeds. Our task, as those who have been designated, appointed, or are dedicated to work with violent youth, is to find the "good" in all youth. Utilizing the VCR approach is one of the cornerstones to counteracting devaluation. At its core, the VCR approach is principally concerned with restoring value. By value, we refer to those attributes that are central to our humanity and sense of self as human beings. Once one's sense of dignity, respect, and personal worth has been assaulted or depleted, the process of restoring is often very slow for all involved.

The Three Steps of the VCR Approach

The VCR approach consists of three steps. Briefly stated, the first step involves validating, which is followed by the second step, challenging or confronting. The successful implementation of these steps paves the way for the final step, requesting.

Step 1: "V" for Validation

Validation means that whatever adolescents say or do, first, before anything else, they need to be validated. This means sending a message that conveys "I understand your perspective—I recognize where you're coming from." Validation consists of sending a message that acknowledges a strength or a goodness in the young person in question. It is important to note that validation is not synonymous with agreement. It is entirely possible to validate someone's perspective without agreeing with it. Validation consists of sending the message "I understand," which is not the same as saying "I agree." One can understand a certain point of view without agreeing with it. By recognizing this critical distinction, it becomes much easier to offer validation.

Step 2: "C" for Challenging

After adults have appropriately and adequately validated adolescents, it then becomes possible to challenge all those troubling teen thoughts and/or behaviors. Moreover, adults who started with the "V" buy themselves a few chips that they can now cash in during the transition into challenging/confronting. However, it is important to point out that how one challenges/confronts is critical. Effective challenging does not and absolutely should not assault the humanity of the adolescent in question. It is possible and necessary for the challenging to happen in a way that preserves the dignity of the adolescent. In fact, the most effective form of challenging weaves in and builds upon the earlier messages of validation. With Timothy, one aspect of our validations of him focused around what a strong leader he was, how smart he was, and how deeply loyal he was to his friends. When we were finally ready to move to the C we softly challenged his cruelty toward his brother, pointing out that he was the type of person who stuck by friends even when they let him down and even when they irritated him. Because he knew his friends looked up to him, and because he was a good leader, he didn't give up on them. He was loyal and patient, and yet how sad it was that he was unable to extend the same loyalty and patience to his own brother. We pointed out how sad it was that he could give more loyalty to his friends than to his own flesh and blood.

Step 3: "R" is for Requesting

After validating and challenging, the third and final step of the VCR approach involves making a request. Here is where the greatest corrective opportunity exists. This stage of the approach allows adolescents to translate the feedback they've received into positive, concrete action. This is especially important in terms of counteracting devaluation, because this last stage allows adolescents to feel some hope about their potential to do things in a more positive way. With Timothy, we wondered if there was any way he could relate to his brother by using the same loyalty, patience, and good leadership skills he used with his friends. We acknowledged that, like his friends, Robert was annoying and sometimes pissed him off. But also, like them, Robert revered him, and needed someone like Timothy to show him the way. We wondered if Timothy could show at least as much loyalty and patience toward his blood brother as he did with his friends. That was our request of him, and this request was very much grounded in a combination of the validating and challenging messages we had presented Timothy with over the course of several weeks.

Guiding Principles for Using The VCR Approach

The VCR is predicated on several essential principles that facilitate its use. These guiding principles provide a framework for how we use the VCR in our work with violent youth. The principles are as follows:

1. *The process of validation must precede any form of challenge or confrontation.* When working with angry, aggressive, and violent youth, one has neither the right nor the license to challenge, confront, or criticize an adolescent until he or she has been appropriately and adequately validated. As a society, we seem to be more adept at giving, receiving, and defending criticism than we are at giving and receiving affirmation. We see this repeatedly in therapy, where it seems far easier for a parent to express criticism of a teenager than it is to tell him or her something they really appreciate about them. Usually our effort to extract even the most benign act of validation often results in lots of giggling and paralyzing levels of discomfort. We typically hear statements like "She knows what I think!" or " I have told him before in my own way." Interestingly, most youth, while craving validation and affirmation privately, also seem to work exceedingly hard during these moments to distract or discourage their parents from following through with what is often considered our mushy request. It seems too hard and uncomfortable for everyone involved. Thus, it is our belief that in most human interactions, if there is a natural position of default during high-intensity, potentially explosive experiences as well as during calm moments of intimacy, we believe it is toward challenging, confronting, and/or criticizing. Even when there is a not an overt expression of criticism, there is an absence of validation or affirmation. This *natural tendency* is magnified during interactions between adults and violent youth. It is something about the demeanor, voice tone, posturing, and overall behavior of these youth that invite spontaneous challenge and critique by adults.

The purpose of this principle, and the VCR approach in general, is to help us to replace spontaneous challenge/criticism with spontaneous validation in our work with violent and aggressive adolescents. Our premise is that providing validation requires mindfulness and a great deal of practice. We believe giving good, consistent, and authentic validation often involves doing that which is counterintuitive. We believe very strongly that there are no circumstances where it would be necessary to challenge an adolescent prior to offering validation. It is the act of validation, especially where devaluation is prevalent, that ultimately makes a viable challenge or critique possible.

2. *The recipient of the validation (the adolescent), not the dispenser (therapist/adult) determines when it has been sufficient.* In our work with violent youth, we often operate from the perspective that validation is the best possible medication for devaluation. It is validation that gradually restores one's sense of value and worthiness. Thus, it is very dif-

ficult for any one of us, whether as therapist, teacher, or parent to know exactly how much validation is needed to make a difference in the life of an adolescent whose sense of worth has been assaulted. We believe that it is important for those of us working with aggressive and violent adolescents to be relentless dispensers of validation, and to not expect it in return nor get trapped into making independent expert assessments about whether or when we have given enough. We believe that the assessment regarding "how much" and "how often" ultimately should be determined by the adolescent.

Often we are asked, "How will you know when you've validated enough and that it's okay to move on to the 'C' part?" Our response is always "The person receiving the validation determines when it's enough." For some adolescents, only a few validating sentences are necessary before they feel sufficiently acknowledged and safe enough to hear a more challenging message. For others, it may be necessary to hold off on the C messages for weeks, maybe even months. For teens whose sense of devaluation runs especially deep, and who find it exceedingly difficult to trust, much preparation has to be done before they will be at a place where they can absorb and integrate a challenging message. Such teens are so accustomed to hearing only critical remarks that they build a tough defensive wall around themselves as a form of protection against the pain of criticism. Whenever an adult speaks to them, they assume it will be a C message, so they quickly move to "tune out." In such cases it may take weeks before a teen starts to relax and trust the validation. But when the teen eventually begins to trust the affirmation, he or she will begin to send cues indicating that they could tolerate hearing a C message.

As a general rule, we believe that one should continue to validate as long as the adolescent responds with a challenge—an act of defiance, volatility, or apathy. When the basic interpersonal posture of the adolescent remains rigidly fixed, we interpret this as an invitation for more validation. Ironically, it has been our experience that most therapists find this very difficult to do. The more hostile, defensive, or uncooperative the adolescent behaves, the more likely the therapist is to either not validate him or her or to do so but withdraw the validation prematurely. This is a trap that many parents fall prey to as well. After parents are painstakingly convinced to try validating their adolescents more, it is very difficult for them to sustain it. We are told over and over again, "I tried it and it didn't work!" Actually it doesn't work when *any* of us validate, expect immediate behavioral change, and then resort to challenging and criticizing. For any child, regardless of age, who has been profoundly devalued, it may take repeated acts of validation in the face of some fairly horrific behavior before a challenge of any magnitude can be received. These are the situations where it becomes extremely useful for us to keep the PTA rule uppermost in mind.

3. *The validation, challenge, and request messages must all be centered around the same topic or theme.* When validation is given in response to one behavior and followed by a challenge directed at an unrelated issue, it undermines the VCR approach and efforts to counteract devaluation. The unattached challenge often invalidates the validating message. Generally, when the focal points, or subjects, of the validation, challenge, and request are disconnected from one another, it makes the validation appear insincere. Any challenge that is not properly buttressed by strong and authentic validation is prone to being perceived as nothing more than an unwarranted criticism or a personal attack. We have found that one of the most effective ways to chisel away at devaluation is to take a strength-based approach that accentuates the positive attributes of an adolescent. Once these are embraced, it makes it a lot easier to encourage the adolescent to see how a given behavior can be both a strength and a weakness. The following vignette from a group therapy session with violent youth offers an example of this principle.

This was the first session following the drive-by shooting of Brian's best friend, Kevin (who was not a client). Appearing a bit solemn, distraught, and generally overcome with emotion, Brian could only access and express anger and outrage. He sat quietly but appeared restless. Staring at the ceiling in a trance-like state, he seemed ready to explode. After sitting for almost a half-hour, he finally broke his silence after he was asked by one of us to share his thoughts and feelings with the group.

> BRIAN: I know all y'all know what went down last week . . . It's totally messed up, man.

There was an unusually eerie silence that pervaded the room, although several group members nodded affirmatively, conveying to Brian that they had heard the news. After a few moments of silence, Brian began to speak again. It was unclear whether he was speaking to the group directly or whether his thoughts were escaping through his lips unbeknownst to him. His words were slow, rhythmic, but cold and raw.

BRIAN: But that's allright 'cause we know who did da' shit and there will be a price for somebody to pay . . . I guarantee you that! Somebody gots to show these punk ass hoes that we mean business . . . Where I come from, I believe in an eye for an eye . . . I'll show them that we ain't gonna be played and that two can play this game.

Brian's comments were loaded and were stated with a chilling sense of calm and resolution. We were very concerned about the potential for violence. Our thoughts and worries were magnified by the fact that several members of the group seem to have subtly and nonverbally reinforced Brian's apparent thirst for revenge.

THERAPIST (KVH): Brian, I am sorry about Aaron's death . . . I know that the two of you were pretty tight. I really appreciate how honest and open you have been with us here today. You have said a lot of very powerful things that brought goose pimples to my body. I know that Aaron would be happy to know that he meant so much to you and that you got his back. I mean, it sounds like you want to stand up for him . . . protect his honor as a loyal and dedicated partner.

BRIAN: It wasn't no damn death . . . it was straight up, cold-blooded murder. That's what it was, *murder*, and there ain't no other way to look at it.

Brian was right. It was murder. Although the therapist said a lot, the use of the word "death" instead of "murder" seemed to have made it difficult for Brian to hear anything else. In some ways, the therapist's feedback had the unintended consequence of aggravating Brian's sense of agitation and rage.

THERAPIST: You are absolutely right, Brian. It was murder and I should have stated that, I am sorry. Even though I screwed up with my words, I am blown away by your undying commitment to Aaron. I think your loyalty as a friend is incredible. I totally understand how and why your loyalty would make you want to get revenge . . . to hurt or pay back those who are responsible for murdering your friend.

Brian didn't say a word as he sat motionless. The veil of sadness that hung over his face was getting more difficult for him to conceal or conquer.

> THERAPIST: I thought when you correctly pointed out to me how my use of the word "death" probably dissed Aaron in a way, was again the action of a loyal friend seeking justice. I admire that about you.

Brian continued to sit without uttering a single word. He did manage to force a very partially developed smile in response to the therapist's statement "I admire that about you."

> THERAPIST: I see you as a courageous and loyal friend. Those traits are really important to me as well. I would feel lucky to have a friend like you who would be so willing to have my back. And yet, I am really worried. I am worried that you will be loyal to Aaron in a way that will require you to be disloyal to yourself and maybe others who feel about you the way you feel about Aaron.
>
> BRIAN: I'm not feelin' you, Doc! I don't know what you are saying?
>
> THERAPIST: Well, it's like when I messed up with the stupid "death" comment . . . you stopped me, made sure I got it right for Aaron and you didn't use your hands, or a piece. That's what I am saying. You were loyal to your loyalty . . . you made sure I did the right thing, and you didn't have to hurt or dis yourself in the process. That's what I am talking about. Are you feelin' me?

There are several points that are noteworthy in this truncated description of the interaction with Brian. However, we will limit our discussion to the points that are most germane to the principle regarding the importance of the V and C messages focusing on the same theme. Throughout the interaction with Brian, the therapist chose to focus on loyalty as an attribute. It is also worth noting here that at no time during the interaction did Brian ever challenge or refute the notion that he was loyal, or that this was anything but an admirable trait to possess. The therapist's view of Brian as someone who was fiercely loyal was consistent with Brain's view of himself. Once there was consensus between Brian and the therapist, moving to the challenge message became a little easier. In essence, Brian was praised for his tremendous loyalty while simultaneously encouraged to critically examine the ways in which it also obscured his judgment.

4. *"And"—in lieu of "but"—and "I messages" are important communication techniques to use to increase effectiveness of the VCR.* The transition from validation to challenge can be a difficult and delicate one. We believe that the transition can be greatly facilitated by using "and" as the connector between the validating message and the challenge. For example, "I think it is great that you are such a loyal friend, and I am worried that your loyalty is going to lead you do something that will get you into a lot of big trouble. I really don't want that to happen to you" When "but" is used as the connector between a validating message and a challenge, it inadvertently negates the validation—such as "I think it's great that you are such a loyal friend *but* I don't want you get into a lot of big trouble. I really don't want that to happen to you." The subtle distinctions between these two statements are significant. In our view, the second message, in a very understated way, either undercuts or completely negates the significance of the loyalty issue. This does not occur with the first message.

In addition to using "and," we believe the use of "I messages" are also vital to effective implementation of the VCR. The effectiveness of using "I messages" has been well documented in the literature (Nunnally & Moy, 1989). For the sake of a quick review, "I messages" in human communication are important because they facilitate the speaker being transparent about his or her thoughts, feelings, wishes, or nonwishes. In this regard, "I messages" enable the speaker to avoid using "you" messages, which essentially leave the listener feeling blamed or criticized. The use of "I" messages is critical to VCR because they help to fortify validating messages.

5. *Avoid asking questions, especially in cases involving high levels of anger and rage.* The VCR works best when feedback is interpreted and shared. We try to avoid, at all costs, asking questions, because they tend to be exceedingly problematic. Questions tend to alter the course of interactions with adolescents in unhealthy and nonfunctional ways. The major problem with questions is twofold. The first difficulty is that questions, especially those asked by therapists and other human service providers, are often disguised challenges. When questions serve this purpose they become a little lethal because they fail to make the therapist's views and opinions clear in a way that communicates

and engenders respect. The response is often extreme guardedness or defensiveness. Secondly, adolescents tend to interpret all questions from adults as challenges, no matter how low-key or innocent they seem to you. It has been our experience that even adolescents who have had no brushes with the law or flirtations with violence detest having to answer questions. With violent youth, we have not found anything that incites anger, rage, or reactive withdrawal from interactions as quickly as does the asking of questions.

EXAMPLES OF THE VCR IN ACTION

Joey

During a routine school consultation at a high school we spent several weeks conducting classroom observations. On one of these days, we found ourselves in a 10th-grade English class where the teacher, Ms. Roundi, was presenting a lecture on the play "Julius Caesar." Mrs. Roundi had been discussing the scene in which members of the Senate, led by Brutus, turn on Caesar and brutally assassinate him. She asked several questions related to this scene. Several students raised their hands, and Ms. Roundi called on them to answer. This pattern persisted, but all the while we noticed that there was one boy, Joey, who, despite eagerly extending his hand, was never called upon. Finally, Ms. Roundi asked, "What do you think about the course of action Brutus took?" Unable to contain himself any longer, Joey shouted out, "I think he's an asshole, and he should be taken to the Coliseum and chopped up alive into little pieces and fed to the lions." Immediately the class burst into laughter, and Joey looked quite pleased with himself. Clearly he reveled in the affirmation of his classmates' laughter. Unfortunately, Ms. Roundi was not nearly as amused. In fact, her expression was one of shock and anger. Seemingly disgusted by Joey's profanity, impulsivity, and graphic statement, she shot back, her eyes blazing, "Joey, I am offended! I do not appreciate your outburst or your foul mouth, and your making comedy out of violence."

Suddenly the twinkle in Joey's eyes was gone. After slumping slightly in his chair, he shrugged his shoulders and then he giggled. But it was an uneasy, half-hearted giggle, the kind people make when they're trying to save face, the type of giggle that's supposed to say "This isn't bothering me, it's funny." But it was clear that it bothered him.

We share this story because it provides a wonderful "teaching moment." As observers of this incident, we agreed with the teacher that Joey's outburst was inappropriate. We also believe he needed some type of corrective intervention from Ms. Roundi. But where we differ from Ms. Roundi is with respect to *how* we believe this intervention should have occurred. From our perspective, she would have been more effective had she employed the VCR approach. Had she opted to do this, she might have responded to Joey in the following way.

1. V: "Joey, I can see that you're eager to participate. I really appreciate your enthusiasm and your willingness to get involved. This is wonderful. It also sounds like what Brutus did really bothers you, and you think he should be punished for that."

2. C: "Even though I know you're really excited about participating, I do need you to wait until I call upon you to speak. Also, while I love that this topic has really got you worked up, and you have some very creative ideas about what should happen to Brutus, I'm not comfortable with your using profanity in the classroom."

3. R: "So, what I would like from you is to please hold on to all that enthusiasm that you have, and next time could you please raise your hand and wait until I call on you, even if it seems like a long time. Also, I am intrigued that you proposed a violent solution for dealing with violence. This would be a good topic to further explore, so I want to ask you to lead the class in a discussion about when and if violence is ever justified."

If Ms. Roundi had engaged Joey using the VCR approach, we believe she could have successfully intervened and redirected him, but more importantly she would have avoided the devaluation that Joey clearly experienced in that moment. It also is important to share that in this particular classroom Ms. Roundi and about two-thirds of the students were white, while the remaining third, including Joey, was African American. This piece of the context is critical, because we believe the racial dynamics in the room contributed to the interaction that unfolded and the effect it had on Joey, in particular. While we can never know this, we believe that to some extent Joey's apparent invisibility to Mrs. Roundi—that is, until he did something wrong—was influenced by the fact that she was white and he was African American. It was rather amazing the number of times Joey's raised hand went unnoticed while several other students, all of whom were white, were acknowledged. It would be impossible to argue that she did not see him, as he was sitting almost directly in front of her. So, why was it so hard for her to really "see" Joey? Why did he remain so invisible despite his obvious visibility? And why is it that Joey was only able to capture her attention once he acted out? How many children every day in our homes and schools struggle with the same dynamic of going virtually unnoticed until they act out, at which point they are labeled "bad kids" (conduct-disordered) or "sick kids" (those with attention-deficit disorder)?

Given the disproportionate number of African American students in comparison to white students who are diagnosed with conduct disorder, attention-deficit/hyperactivity disorder (ADHD), or some type of learning disability, it seems hard to dismiss racial bias as an intervening variable. But, even if we gave Ms. Roundi the benefit of the doubt and conceded that race was not an organizing principle in her treatment of Joey, even still, race was significant to Joey. In several conversations we had with Joey, it was clear to us that he was aware of the fact that he was an African American in a predominantly white school. Moreover, he already harbored decisive feelings about how he often felt alienated and rejected as a black person. So, when Joey was publicly scorned by his teacher, part of him was experiencing this as an African American youth in front of his mostly white class and white teacher. Not only had Joey been devalued as an individual, but here was yet one more instance in his young life where he was devalued as a black person in a white world. Even if race had not been an organizing principle in Ms Roundi's treatment of Joey, shouldn't it have been? Should she not have had enough racial sensitivity to realize, in spite of her own intentions, how sensitive Joey might have been to any criticism or shame as one of the few black kids in this largely white classroom?

Bobby

Mr. Valoz had two sons, Bobby, 13, and Peter, 11. Father and sons were sitting together in their family room one Sunday afternoon. Mr. Valoz was watching TV, and the two boys were playing on the computer on the other side of the room. Mr. Santos just happened to glance over in the direction of the boys in time to observe Bobby punching Peter, who started to cry. Mr. Valoz intervened and asked Bobby why he had hit Peter. "Because he took another turn on the game, and it was my turn," Bobby replied. To his credit, Mr. Valoz first responded to Bobby by validating him.

1. V: Mr. Valoz said to Bobby, "Well that wasn't very nice of Peter. I'm sure that must have made you mad. I know how important fairness is to you, and that you think it's very important for people to treat each other with consideration. I can understand why you would be upset at Peter for doing something that must have seemed so inconsiderate and unfair."

Mr. Valoz was validating Bobby for his perspective. He was letting Bobby know that he understood his point of view, and he was acknowledging one of Bobby's strengths, namely, his strong sense of integrity and commitment to fairness and consideration. The value in his validation is that it allowed Bobby to feel understood, and it helped him to trust that his father could see something good in him.

After having validated Bobby, thereby putting him at ease and gaining a piece of trust, Mr. Santos was in a better position to challenge him.

2. C: Mr. Valoz challenged Bobby in the following way: "It's not considerate to take something that's not yours. It's also not considerate to hit and punch other people. It just makes me sad that the way you chose to teach Peter a lesson was by being inconsiderate and unfair back to him. It's just that I know that's not the type of person you are."

While Mr. Valoz presented Bobby with a challenge, he was careful to do it gently, in a way that allowed him to retain a piece of dignity. This is a critical point. Often, when we endeavor to train people in the use of the VCR approach, they assume that once they have validated, this gives them license to be brutal when they get to the challenging part. Unfortunately, this assumption can be very damaging. The main function of validation is to earn a little piece of trust and provide a foundation for restoring value. If an adult is able to secure this trust through validation, it becomes a tragic miscalculation to follow up by then slamming the adolescent with a harshly critical message. Instead, the challenge must be carefully presented in such a way that it preserves, rather than assaults, the humanity of the person is question.

Having validated and challenged, Mr. Valoz completed the VCR approach by making a request of Bobby.

3. R: Mr. Valoz made the following request: "Because I know you are a considerate and fair person, and that you're very smart, I bet you could have thought of other ways to teach Peter that what he did wasn't very nice. In fact, let's think now of three ways you could have done this without hitting and punching."

Hence, Mr. Valoz sent Bobby a powerful message that he viewed him as a considerate, intelligent person who was committed to fairness. He also let him know that in this case, unfortunately, he may have betrayed his own principles when he hit Peter. Finally, he gave him an opportunity to "right his wrong" by using his sense of fairness, consideration, and intelligence to explore alternative ways of responding to Peter that would allow Bobby to remain true to his ideals.

Jason

When we first met Jason, it was like déjà vu. Jason, who was 15 at the time, had suffered the loss of his best friend, Hank. In a gang-related incident, Hank had been shot to death; he'd been hit with three bullets in the chest and one in the head. Jason and Hank had been extremely close friends since third grade. Now, after his tragic loss, Jason was obsessed with revenge: "I know the punk who took Hank out, and you can best believe he's gonna get what's coming to him for what he did." Interestingly, Jason was in the same therapy group with Brian (whom we referred to earlier in this chapter). In many ways, their lives were mirror images of each other. Tracey was the lead therapist for this session. It was our very first session together. Our instincts told us that his comment was referring to something extreme, so we probed further to get clarification about what he was planning.

"Hey, he smoked Hank, so he's gonna get the same. I owe it to Hank. He's never gonna get to do everything he dreamed of. Never. And that is so wrong. If it's the last thing I do, I'm gonna do right by him." Jason was determined to live by what he referred to as "Jason's golden rule": "do unto others as they have done to you." A rival gang member had taken out his best friend's life, and Jason was gonna' strike back and take the life of Hank's murderer. Hearing the resolve in Jason's voice was unnerving. It certainly sent a chill up our spines, because we could see from the hardened, unflinching expression on Jason's face that his threats were more than rhetorical—he meant what he was saying. We desperately wanted to stop Jason from following through with his deadly revenge, but we also realized that how we responded to him was critical. We also understood that an obsession with revenge is a common reaction of adolescents who have lost loved ones to random violence. This reaction is so commonplace that we not only expect it but also consider it a fundamental part of the grieving process for violent youth.

Every fiber in our bodies was screaming at us to jump in and quickly reprimand him for even considering such a senseless and brutal reaction to Hank's death. We wanted to point out to him that revenge wouldn't bring Hank back and that most likely it would only result in further violence and/or his incarceration. We wanted him to see the pointlessness of striking back. We wanted him to exercise saner, more rational, judgment. And if he wouldn't listen to reason or to our impassioned plea, we wanted to scream at him and berate him into listening to us. And yet, despite our strongest desire to respond like this, we also had learned along the way that such approaches rarely, if ever, produce the desired result. Instead, we knew that Jason would merely tune us out, write us off as clueless adults who simply could not understand. He would feel misunderstood and alienated by such an approach. Yet, we also knew we had to find some way to deter him from exacting his revenge. Consequently, we used the VCR approach.

1. V: I (TAL) began by saying to Jason, "I can really see how much you loved Hank and how close the two of you were. We can't even begin to imagine how intense your loss and pain must be. I know you probably feel like you have to hold it all together now and be strong. Seeing how much you obviously loved him, you must really be hurting inside. I can also see that Hank was lucky to have you as a friend. Obviously you are a deeply loyal friend. It's hard to come by true friends—those who love you enough that they would risk their own lives for you. It seemed like you and Hank had that type of special bond, and we really admire your devotion to your friend. And because you loved him so much and must be really hurting over his loss, I can understand why you would feel compelled to want to remain loyal to Hank even in death. It makes sense that you would want to strike back against the person who hurt him and hurt you."

As my comments revealed, my initial approach with Jason was focused solely around validation. I validated the significance of his relationship with Hank and the pain he must have been feeling in response to his loss. I also validated Jason for being a loyal friend. The hardest part of my validation involved conveying that I understood why he would want to kill the young man who murdered Hank. But even as I conveyed understanding for Jason's perspective, the careful observer will recognize that my message was not one of condoning violence. I never agreed that committing murder was the right thing to do; I only expressed that we (obviously speaking for Ken) could understand why he would want to take this course of action. I expressed understanding for his feelings.

After spending a sufficient amount of time with Jason validating his feelings and his perspective, the next step was to move toward challenging him.

> 2. C: I challenged him by saying: "I know how important loyalty is to you, and how devoted you were and still are to Hank. After all, if you take out this other guy, his buddies will probably have to do the same to you. I know your commitment to Hank is so strong you would sacrifice yourself. I do not doubt your willingness to die for him—I just doubt whether it's the best way to honor him. After all, if you die, Hank will die with you. No one knew him like you did, and no one understood his dreams like you did. If you die there will be no one to carry on for him."

Our method in challenging Jason involved building upon the very qualities and points we had identified and emphasized when we were simply validating him. I tried to use a frame that was meaningful to Jason, namely, one of loyalty, friendship, sacrifice, and brotherhood. Some of these same themes were highlighted with Brian, who also had an insatiable thirst for revenge. I tried to take the things that were important to Jason and give him a different way of thinking about them, one that would challenge his current thinking about the best way to respond to the tragic loss of his friend.

Finally, I made a request of Jason that wove together the validating and the challenging parts of my message to him.

> 3. R: I made the following request: "I know the most important thing to you is being loyal to Hank, and we know you have the courage to die for him. I hope that you have enough courage to live for him. I hope there is a way you could find the strength to resist the temptation of striking back violently and instead

commit your energy toward doing the things Hank was never able to do for himself. Could you carry on in his honor, in his footsteps, so his life won't be truly lost forever? I know it's a harder path to take because it doesn't have a quick 'payoff' or sense of immediate gratification, but could you love Hank enough to hang in there and deal with the tougher path for his sake?"

What I attempted to accomplish with this last stage in the VCR approach was to make a request of Jason that oriented him toward something concrete that he could do to fulfill both his need and my need for him. Hence, I asked him if he could find a way to resist revenge as a way of showing his loyalty. I asked him if he could explore a different way of showing his love, one that would allow him to keep the memory of his dear friend alive. So far, Jason has managed to stay violence-free.

Lena

Lena had been sexually abused by her stepfather from the age of 6 to 13. At that point her mother divorced her stepfather, and at last the abuse ended. But Lena's trauma wounds remained raw. The shame of the abuse had inflicted a deep sense of profound devaluation. She stated, "I feel like I am the most disgraceful, worthless human being alive. I wish I could just crawl out of my skin and never have to look myself in the mirror again." The abuse also had disrupted her sense of community at the primary level, because it left her feeling as if "home" was not a safe place. Moreover, because she feared her mother's reaction, she kept the abuse a secret. At the extended community level, Lena's stepfather, who was deeply controlling and possessive, discouraged her from socializing with friends. In a way Lena didn't object because she often felt uncomfortable around other kids, fearful that if she got too close to friends they might be able to see how disgraceful she was. Because no one knew about the abuse (or at least, no one acknowledged knowing), Lena's pain and loss were unacknowledged, which meant her loss essentially had been dehumanized.

When Lena was 14, the school nurse had noticed suspicious scars on her legs. They appeared to be cuts that had been inflicted by a knife or a razor. When the nurse first asked about the cuts, Lena said she didn't know how she had gotten them. The nurse was suspicious and gently persisted until eventually Lena confessed that she had inflicted the wounds herself. The nurse realized that Lena needed help, so she referred her to the school psychologist, who consulted with me (TAL) on this case.

Eventually Lena confessed the abuse and explained to the psychologist that "I cut myself because it helps to relieve the hurt I feel inside. It's like a moment of relief when it all just oozes out. I have to do this, or else I don't know what I would do. I might go crazy otherwise. I would lose it, and I can't let that happen, because I don't want my mom to be upset. She has suffered enough. Please, you can't tell my mom about this."

Lena was a clear example of a young person who had internalized her rage that had been transformed into violence against herself. She elected to target herself rather than directing her violence outwardly, because she believed this would be the least selfish way of handling her emotions. The psychologist employed the VCR in her work with Lena.

1. V: The psychologist said to Lena, "I find it amazing how after all that you have suffered you still find a way to care about others. It's moving to see how much you love your mom, even to the point that you would choose to suffer alone rather than see your mom suffer. In addition to your willingness to make sacrifices for your mom, it also is clear to me that you are very strong. It's got to take a lot of strength to have survived your stepfather's abuse, and to endure your pain now in silence."

The psychologist was affirming Lena for her love and commitment to her mother and her strength with regard to her ability to make sacrifices and endure suffering if she believed it was for the sake of others.

2. C: The psychologist went on to challenge Lena by stating, "I really appreciate all the effort that you are willing to make in order to protect your mother, and I am thinking that keeping things from her won't feel like protection to her if she ever finds out. I am scared and worried because cutting yourself is very dangerous. You could end up doing a lot of damage, and then imagine how your mom would feel." I went on to further challenge Lena ever so gently by suggesting, "I am imagining that there might be other ways to protect your mom besides hurting yourself, although it's possible that these other ways might seem harder at first. But then again, you've proven that

you're very strong and that you are willing to face hardships if it means protecting those you love."

The psychologist was using the attributes she had used to validate Lena to also challenge her. First, she softly challenged Lena's decisions by expressing doubt that her chosen course of action was the best way to protect her mom. She then suggested that if Lena wanted to protect her mother, maybe there was another way, a more effective way, of accomplishing this. She also drew upon the validation she had offered Lena about her strength, especially when it came to making sacrifices for others, so she could advance a challenge. Essentially, she proposed that there might be a better way for Lena to protect her mother, although it might be harder for her. And yet, since it already had been established that Lena was strong, and could be especially strong if it meant protecting her mother, she would probably be able employ one of these other, more effective, methods even if it were more difficult initially.

3. R: The psychologist made the following request: "Even though this may seem harder, I think the best way to protect your mom is to be sure that nothing worse happens to you and to make sure that you will be okay. I think you need to do this for your mom's sake. I know this is going to be really hard for you, but you've proven how strong you can be, especially when it comes to making sacrifices for your mom. So, I am going to ask you make a sacrifice here and tell your mom what has happened so that you can give her a chance to feel like a good mom by letting her help you. At the same time, it's going to mean that we need to find another way for you to relieve your hurting. For now, whenever you think you need to cut yourself, you can come see me instead, or call me, or you can write me a note. I will give you these red envelopes, and any time you write me a note telling me about the hurt, I want you to seal it in one of these envelopes and mail it to me . . . in other words, I want you to send it off . . . send off the hurt and send it out and away from you. Let me hold it for you for now."

In this way, the psychologist was giving Lena something specific and concrete that she could do to address her pain and suffering and to still protect and care for her mother. She accomplished this by building upon the initial qualities in Lena that had been validated.

The Challenges of Validating

There are a number of challenges that make it especially difficult for adults to validate adolescents. First, validation is often confused with agreement. Thus, there seems to be an understandable and pervasive fear that, if a questionable position or act of an adolescent is validated, this is tantamount to condoning it. We believe that it is possible to understand someone's position without necessarily agreeing with it. For example, saying "I can understand why you want to punch him out—I think you have a right to feel angry" is not the same as encouraging the behavior. This message is one of validation, *not* agreement. Nowhere in the message is the speaker condoning punching. However, there is an acknowledgment of understanding regarding why one might want to do this. Once this distinction is recognized, the easier it becomes to validate.

Second, many of us find it difficult to validate adolescents because of our own reactivity to the things they say and do. On the milder side, many of us simply feel irritated by typical adolescent antics. On the more threatening side, some of us are overwhelmed by fear in response to the thoughts and behaviors some adolescents manifest. Our feelings of worry and fear are heightened when we are working with aggressive and violent youth. Their threatened or actual violence strikes a panic chord within us that not only compels us to react but frequently dictates how we react as well. In our experience, panic-driven reactions, more often than not, tend to be defensive responses that are counterproductive. Whether the panic-driven, defensive response is retaliatory, thus leading to an escalating sequence of attack–counterattack, or withdrawal that is the impetus for reactive cutoff, in either case meaningful effective communication is blocked.

When adolescents engage in ways of thinking and behaving that involve threatened or actual violence, it is imperative to closely monitor and manage our panic-driven, defensive reactions. Failure to do so only invites comparably defensive responses from the adolescents with whom we are interacting. In accordance with the adolescent axioms (see Chapter 6), those of us working with adolescents must be stronger and healthier than those with whom we interact. This means we have to be able to work around our own instinctual impulses—to develop the type of inner fortitude that will enable us to act rather than react. The ability to validate—even when faced with the most heinous and disturbing of circumstances—is deeply rooted in this inner fortitude. It requires enormous inner control and strength to respond in a validating way to an adolescent who is involved in threatened or actual violence. The concern, anxiety, and fear that we may feel in such instances often compels many of us to quickly intervene by using the C's. Unfortunately, because the C's tend to alienate adolescents and aggravate devaluation, we instantly undermine our own objective. Counteracting devaluation requires putting the C's in "pause" mode while we validate, validate, and validate.

A third challenge that often makes validation difficult is when validation is delivered in a way that appears insincere or when it is used primarily as a technique. For validation to be effective, the dispenser (the person offering it) must be sincere and the feedback authentic. This is why earlier in this chapter we suggested that the VCR is more than a clinical technique. It is as much a way of looking at the world as it is a strategy or technique. It is difficult to affirm the good attributes of bad kids if you don't believe the former exist. Thus, if a validating message is contrived, the receiver will realize this, and the spirit underlying the validation will be thwarted. Adolescents who are aggressive and violent are also among the most devalued, and they are exceedingly sensitive to, as they would call it, "being played," or made to look stupid. When a validating message is stated insincerely, or is too sterile and clinical, adolescents tend to feel manipulated. I believe the first critical step to mastering validation is to change what we look for so that we can change what we see. If we look for pearls of goodness entangled in badness, we are very likely to find the good. If, on the other hand, we are limited to looking for badness, it is undoubtedly what we ultimately see.

As youth violence has been thrust to the forefront of society, one of the major societal responses to the epidemic has been to get tougher with (bad) kids. In the past several years we have seen the proliferation of "zero tolerance" programs in schools, an increasing number of middle school children tried as adults in the criminal justice system, as well as a host of other initiatives designed to get tougher. Consequently, as a society, our dominant response to youth who commit almost any type of transgression, minor or major, is punishment. Whether it's the third grader who has just cheated on a quiz, the 13-year-old who just got caught drinking a six-pack with her best friend, or the 17-year-old who just robbed and beat a woman who was walking to her car in a parking lot. In each of these cases we have children and adolescents behaving badly. Feeling a sense of outrage, dismay, and grave worry in response to each of these incidents is understandable. Unfortunately, however, as a society we seem hopelessly stuck in our instinctive desire to punish young people like these for their transgressions. We believe that the *orientation toward punishment* makes validation tough to implement. It is very difficult to validate a violent youth when we are increasingly oriented toward punishment. Consequently, we shame, shun, label, lock up, lock down, isolate, alienate, berate, and banish those who defy our codes of morality and laws of order.

Whenever we conduct workshops on the orientation toward punishment, we inevitably get the attention of those who believe that our seeming unwillingness to hold bad kids "accountable" is *precisely* what has gone wrong with today's youth. They are always worried that the tenor of our comments regarding punishment is a pitch for sentimental, bleeding-heart liberalism. To the contrary, the point we wish to make is that when kids act up and act out, if our only response is punishment, we do very little to improve much of anything. Consider for a moment what the purpose of punishment is—namely, to make sure than the perpetrator of an offense *suffers*. Ironically, our orientation toward punishment is not fundamentally different from Brian and Jason's desire to exact revenge upon the perpetrators who killed their best friends. The goal appears to be to make perpetrators *hurt* for their crimes rather than to *repair the damage* that led to the crime in the first place.

According to James Garbarino (1999), an expert in the area of youth violence:

> The greatest danger comes when the crisis of perceived impending psychic annihilation is melodramatically merged with the idea of addressing intolerable injustice with violence. The two go together, because in our society the idea of retribution through violence is a basic article of faith. Vengeance is not confined to some small group of psychologically devastated individuals. It is normal for us. A fact of value in our culture. (p. 133)

Garbarino is challenging us to recognize several critical points. First, he reminds us that much of the violence adolescents commit is a response to some injustice that they perceive—injustices that are intolerable to them. Second, Garbarino is asserting that, as a society, we are no different from these kids (even though most of us claim not to understand them). We, like them, believe in retribution through violence. When we feel we are the victims of an injustice, we too support the use of violence as a means of coping with our pain. Is this not the basic underlying message associated with the death penalty, or our response to the September 11 acts of terrorism? Hence, as individuals and as a society, we need to recognize our own hypocrisy with respect to how we respond to adolescent violence. While it may be true that the so-called injustices that provoke many adolescents to violence hardly seem justified to reasonable people, nonetheless the model they are using to respond to their pain is one that we have taught them. It's a model that some of us defend ardently even while we claim not to understand adolescents who become violent.

Moreover, some critical reevaluating of the punishment model that we rely on to deal with injustice and pain is crucial. When we use brutal methods to deal with violent teens, we betray ourselves in so many ways. Punishment may feel good to us (just as it feels good to teens who use aggression to strike back at their tormentors), but it does very little to counteract devaluation, or to promote positive change and healing. By relying solely on punishment as our dominant response to violent youth, we merely reinforce rather than reform their violence. In a perverse twist of irony, we become the embodiment of the very thing we are punishing them for.

Validation through Giving

One of the great misconceptions that exist about validation is that it is achieved primarily through receiving. While it may indeed be validating to be the recipient of gifts, kind words, loving gestures, and other types of positive commodities, the greatest form of validation is achieved through the act of giving. When people have something to give, they are validated in the highest way. Having something meaningful to offer others, something that others regard as a valuable commodity, validates the giver in the deepest of ways. Perhaps the major difference between the validation derived from giving versus receiving is that in the case of the former there is a sense of empowerment associated with the "doing" aspect of giving, which stands in contrast to the more passive, potentially disempowering stance associated with receiving. This may in fact help to explain why acts of charity, while benevolently motivated, often leave the receiver feeling ashamed and powerless. At first glance, receiving charity should be validating, because the unstated message is "you are valued enough to warrant this act of kindness." And yet, being in a position of having to rely on others for acts of kindness defines the receiver in a subordinate position to the giver, which ultimately is antithetical to the experience of validation. Hence, it is through having something meaningful to give to others that people experience the greatest form of validation.

In our treatment of violent youth who have been profoundly devalued, we spend an inordinate amount of time deliberately searching for the *gifts of giving* that we believe they inevitably possess. We believe that the process of discovering their gifts of giving is one of the most pivotal moments of therapy, especially with regard to counteracting devaluation.

I (TAL) once saw a young man in therapy named Shariff. At the tender age of 17, he already had been stabbed in the chest (narrowly missing his heart), had his nose broken, and had suffered three cracked ribs and a concussion as a result of numerous altercations with his enraged girlfriend, rival gang members, and a boy at school who had insulted his hair style. Shariff was most at ease when he was involved in some type of fight. Whenever he felt disrespected, no matter how slight, the response was almost always to threaten or act out violently. The more time I spent with Shariff, the more apparent it was that he suffered from a profound sense of devaluation. There had been the rejection in his primary community when his mother abandoned him when he was 10, leaving him with an aunt (he had no idea who his father was). He also had felt devalued at school, where he was labeled learning disabled (not coincidentally also when he was 10, just a few months after his mother's abandonment, but a connection that nonetheless went unrecognized by anyone in his school) and was placed in a special education class that left him feeling "like a stupid idiot." Being biracial (his mother was African American and his father white), he also felt racially devalued by both whites and African Americans. "Most white folks believe that if you have any color in you at all, you're just a nigger, and for most black folks I guess I'm just not black enough." When Shariff was 13, he joined a racially mixed gang, which provided him with the only sense of acceptance and community he had ever known. But even with the gang and in some ways because of it, he suffered with feeling like an outsider. He still carried the pain of his many unhealed losses and the corresponding rage that led him to want to beat up anyone who dared to look at him questioningly.

When Shariff began his court-ordered therapy sessions with me, one of the goals that I knew I had to achieve was to find ways to counteract his sense of devaluation. In spite of all the crazy—even downright disturbing—things he had done, there were ways in which Shariff made it easy for me to validate him. He was extremely bright (which in my opinion certainly called into question the learning disability he had been diagnosed with). I also eventually discovered that he had an amazing knack for troubleshooting electronics equipment. I discovered this one day when one of our video cameras was on the blink. Shariff volunteered to take a look at it, and within minutes he had disassembled portions of it that, from my perspective, seemed amazingly confusing and intricate. But Shariff moved with a grace and confidence that was startling. Within 10 minutes he had fixed the video camera, and we subsequently had no trouble with it at all. We were extremely grateful to him, because we had struggled with this camera for nearly a year, unable to diagnosis or repair it ourselves and too busy to seek out the expertise we needed. And here, in a matter of minutes, our problem had been solved! And quite by chance I had also solved another dilemma I had been struggling with—how to counteract devaluation in Shariff's life. While I knew that Shariff had grown to trust and respect me, I never completely felt that I had been able to penetrate the layers of devaluation that he seemed buried under—that is, until the video camera episode.

After Shariff successfully repaired our video camera, my relationship with him changed profoundly. Suddenly he had something valuable to offer me. Suddenly I was no longer the only one with the expert knowledge. This incident established his expertise in an area where I clearly had none, and it allowed him to give me something we very much needed and appreciated. The pride Shariff felt was evident. He enthusiastically offered to fix anything else that needed to be repaired.

In the case of Shariff, it just so happens that his *gift for giving* involved something very concrete—his practical knowledge of electronics technology. However, most of the gifts for giving that are highlighted in our work are far less tangible. Often they involve unrecognized or untapped personal attributes that are most commonly minimized. For anyone daring to look more deeply at Brian and Jason, the two hot-headed, vengeance-thirsty threats to society, even they had gifts for giving. In each case, these two adolescents possessed the gift of undying loyalty. They were loyal to the point that it gave them something to both live and die for—what a precious gift to have to offer! Our task as their therapists was to identify their capacity for giving and to help them recognize, actualize, and maximize their gifts. Our goal is always to help the Brians and Jasons of society find socially sanctioned vessels for their gifts. After all, it is our view that "giving" denied expression is validation denied.

The power of validation through having something to give has taught us that when working with adolescents, especially those prone to violence, it is extremely helpful to identify their capacity for giving. The giving can be almost anything—teaching a younger brother, sister, or neighborhood child how to improve their jump shots, tutoring a fellow classmate in a favorite subject, sharing the wisdom they gained about how to get out of a gang with other adolescents who are still struggling to get out, helping a parent with a younger sibling or chores around the house, picking up groceries for an elderly relative, volunteering at a nursing home or youth center, or caring for a newly acquired pet. The list of possibilities is limitless. The important thing is to explore the unique strengths and interests of each adolescent. It is our view that any failure to uncover an adolescent's gift is the result of our not looking closely enough, our not seeing all the possibilities, or our not believing strongly enough.

Badges of Ability

Badges and gifts for giving are related but different. We believe that gifts are usually unconscious—or at least they are usually outside of the everyday awareness of most of us. Also, gifts are strengths or attributes that require the act of giving. If a gift is recognized but not given, it may very well be a badge.

Lillian Rubin (1992) developed the concept of "Badges of Ability" in her landmark study of working-class families. Badges of ability are strengths that individuals possesses that they proudly identify and display to the world. It is a positive attribute that they can "pin" on their shirts like a badge for others to observe and validate. As adults who work with adolescents, we believe that it is important for us to be able to identify and validate at least one badge of ability in each and every adolescent with whom we interact. Ideally, we believe it is useful to identify and begin affirming these badges early on in our relationships with these kids to establish a foundation that we can continue to refer to and draw upon throughout our relationship. If we cannot identify a single badge of ability that an adolescent has, we firmly believe we are missing a salient opportunity to connect with and promote that young person's optimal potential. It is worth mentioning that when we talk with adolescents we never use the term "badge of ability." This term is most certainly not very "cool" and hence is likely to be greeted somewhat unfavorably. Hence, while the term provides us with a useful framework to guide our work, when we talk with teens we use phrases such as "a strength of yours" or "one of your special skills or qualities."

As a first step toward identifying badges of ability in adolescents, we recommend asking oneself the following questions about each adolescent one has a relationship with:

1. What is at least one badge of ability that this adolescent has?
2. How can I use this badge to facilitate this person's growth and learning?
3. In what ways can I continue to recognize and validate this badge?
4. What are the possible factors that may be preventing me from identifying at least one badge of ability for this adolescent?

If one is unable to identify a single badge for a particular adolescent, this is usually an important indicator of an area that warrants further attention. Moreover, if one has been remiss in validating and capitalizing upon an identified badge, this is critical (self) feedback as well. We recommend looking closely at self-of-the-therapist factors with regard to all of these issues, because working with violent and aggressive adolescent is a demanding challenge for even the best of us.

Cultural Translators

We believe that those of us who work with children and adolescents have a new role that has been defined by the world we live in today. We live in a confusing society. In a world that is increasingly shaped by technology, terrorism, and trauma, it can prove to be a very difficult place for most young people today to fully grasp. The technological advances of society have helped to create a microwave-age society where the efficacy of what we do is typically measured by the rapidity with which it is accomplished. Our children—even those who have had all of the so-called right experiences—are growing up in a world where they live with a powerful but faceless message that demands everything be done in record speed. As a result, they must learn to talk, walk, date, and marry—all with deliberate *speed*. Their world is one of electronic gadgets and machines—Gameboys, Xboxes, iPods, cell phones, and computers. Playing and interacting with others directly has become as antiquated as the black-and-white television set. The world as we know it, and as young people experience it, is one that is rapidly paced and increasingly impersonalized. We all have become frighteningly proficient at communicating cryptically worded messages via voicemails and e-mails in a nanosecond. Conversation and dialogue—once the centerpiece of relationships—are now skill-based academic courses, while remaining inconspicuously absent from our personal lives. Our world is one in which too many of us live our lives vicariously through myriad "reality shows" that permeate our existence. And, just think: some of us, with righteous indignation, have the audacity to ask, "What is wrong with kids today? . . . They don't seem to care about anything anymore." In our opinion, it is a tough, confusing world for most kids to understand.

Each of us who works with young people today has a moral responsibility to take on the role of cultural translator. This role is one that must be integrated with the capacity in which we interface with the lives of young people, particularly those prone to violence. The cultural translator is an interpreter of cultural norms, conflicts, contradictions, and ambiguities. The complexity and perversity of today's world demands interpretation and deconstruction. In this vein, those of us who are therapists can ill afford to simply see our work as that which deals with the intrapsychic and the interpersonal—we must also wrestle with the cultural. Our therapeutic conversations must be expanded to explore traditionally unexplored territory. It is crucial that we remain curious about potential connections between annihilating quickly moving animated objects in popular videogames and killing other kids, or potential connections between terrorism in society and terrorism in the home. These are merely two examples of what we believe constitute the vast domain of the cultural translator. Above all, we believe that the cultural translator role demands that we, in the words of adolescents, "keep it *real*."

With respect to counteracting devaluation, the role of a cultural translator is to help adolescents deconstruct and resist the countless cultural messages they are exposed to every day that assault their sense of humanity. For example, adults can and should play a central role in helping teens to sort through prejudicial and derogatory messages about underrepresented groups based on race, gender, sexual orientation, class, or religion. As one teen said to us during a consultation we did with at her school: "It's hard being a female, because everywhere you turn people are saying things are better now for women and we've become equal with men. But when I watch TV or look in magazines, or even listen to how boys talk to me, I don't feel very equal. I don't even feel respected. It's still messed up out there being a girl, but everybody seems to be trippin."

This young woman was struggling with the mixed messages she was receiving about gender, and what she desperately needed was an adult who could act as a cultural translator. She needed someone who could affirm her perceptions and assure her she wasn't crazy. She needed someone who could help her appreciate that, while women have made important strides in the past several decades, there is still a long way to go. Most importantly, she needed someone she could talk to about the ways she feels devalued as a female so that she can eventually begin to separate how some people (males) look at and treat her, versus who she actually is. Without the help of a cultural translator, in all likelihood this girl will graduate into adulthood convinced that there is something wrong with her. She will never feel like anything more than just a male plaything, but at the same time she won't feel justified in feeling disrespected or even angry about her sense of devaluation as a woman.

Cultural Transformers

Cultural transformers are people who use their power to challenge broader social conditions that contribute to devaluation. Such persons actively use themselves to resist the forces of racism, sexism, classism, heterosexism/homophobia, and all other "isms" that lead to the systematic denigration and oppression of certain groups within society. If each of us were to assume a position of social activism in this regard, think how radically different our world would be today! Think how much we could accomplish in terms of counteracting the devaluation that so many adolescents today experience by virtue of their membership in a particular racial, gender, sexual orientation, class, or religious group!

CONCLUSION

We have identified several strategies to counteract devaluation in the lives of violent adolescents. The first of these is the VCR approach, which provides adults with a clearly identifiable set of steps they can follow to talk with adolescents about complex and potentially volatile issues. Since the mot immediate antidote for devaluation is validation, the VCR begins by affirming the positive aspects of a teen's behaviors and/or personality. Once the teen accepts the validation, the approach shift to challenging whatever the troublesome behavior or belief is, but even this occurs in a manner that builds upon and reinforces the initial validation. Finally, the VCR ends with a request that enables the teen to translate the feedback he or she has received into some concrete doable action that has the potential to "turn things around." The challenges associated with validating were discussed, and several other strategies for counteracting devaluation were examined, including the use of badges of ability, validation through giving, and roles that adults may assume as cultural translators and cultural transformers.

CHAPTER 8

• • • • • • • •

The Restoration
of Community

"I don't feel like I belong anywhere . . . nowhere."

We looked into Carmen's eyes and could see the isolation and alienation that haunted her. She was tortured by a feeling of disconnectedness that was sucking the life out of her. This disconnectedness was the result of a massive disruption of community at all three levels. Through our therapy with Carmen we had learned about how she had lost her birth parents when she was 6, her ties to the small village she once called home, and all the people who had loved and cared for her as part of her extended community. Even after Carmen was adopted by the Brodys, who adored her, we found out that she could never feel a true sense of community with them as long as they denied her cultural identity. As long as they pretended that she was white, as long as she could never tell them how she was called "Indian nigger" and "Pocahontas" at school, Carmen suffered from the disruption of community at all three levels. But piecing all of this together was just the first step. Next, we had to go about the task of promoting the restoration of community in Carmen's life. It was a task we've had to face with every violent teen we've worked with.

In the following sections we outline specific indicators that parents, therapists, teachers, and other concerned adults can look for to identity the disruption of community in the lives of teens. We also provide concrete strategies and recommendations for how adults can embark upon the difficult task of promoting the restoration of community at the primary, extended, and cultural levels in the lives of adolescents.

PRIMARY COMMUNITY

For adolescents, the most traumatic disruption of the primary community occurs in their relationships with parents. Disruptions at the primary level can occur in relationships with other family members, but because the parent–adolescent bond is usually the most important family relationship, we focus most of our attention here.

Indicators of Disruptions in Parent–Adolescent Relationships

There are some situations where disruptions of parent–adolescent relationships are obvious. For example, when parents and teens have little to no contact with one another, this usually is a symptom of strained relationships. When parents are abusive, again this is an obvious indication of a disruption in the primary community. There are some situations, however, that are harder to recognize. For instance, the disruptions that occur in cases of verbal or emotional abuse and neglect can be difficult to detect.

Identifying disruptions in parent–adolescent relationships is further complicated by the fact that it is normal for parents and teens to argue, and generally they have a hard time getting along. Feelings of bitterness, frustration, and anger are common during this stage of development. In situations that seem ambiguous, the rule that we apply is to try to understand how things seem from the teen's point of view. When teens indicate that they feel both *alienated from* and *rejected by* their parents, we view this as an indication that the parent–adolescent bond has been disrupted.

We use the term "alienated" to mean that teens feel estranged from their parents. They experience a lack of connection with their parents, which is often expressed by references to feeling alone, lonely, and as if their parents don't care or understand how they're feeling. As a result, these teens suffer from emotional isolation and loneliness in relation to their parents. We use the term "rejected" to mean that teens believe the reason for the distance between them and their parents is that their parents have turned away from them. Teens often express this by saying things like "My parents don't like me," or "My mom doesn't want to have anything to do with me," or "My dad can't stand how I am."

We believe the parent–adolescent relationship is of critical importance, and therefore a lot of our work in terms of promoting the restoration of primary community focuses on this relationship. In the following sections we outline several different strategies that parents, therapists, teachers, and other concerned adults can employ to repair relationships at the primary level between parents and adolescents.

How Parents Can Repair Relationships with Their Teens

When disruptions occur in parent–adolescent bonds, we believe parents have the greatest obligation to initiate repairs. We offer several strategies that parents can utilize to achieve these repairs and thereby promote the restoration of community at the primary level. Some of these strategies may be harder to employ than others. Depending upon the level of development and available emotional resources of a family, some parents may be capable of effectively employing these strategies independently. Others may require the assistance of trained professionals (e.g., therapists, parent educators) who can assist them with these strategies and the process of relationship reparation.

Engage in Retrospective Reflections

It seems inevitable that parents, especially during times of tremendous personal strife, will engage in a process of analysis about what went wrong. We have found that one of the factors that separate parents who have success in restoring community from those who don't is in the ability to engage in critical self-analysis. Parents who have the capacity to take a hard look at their lives as parents and as (former) children seem to have an easier time repairing ruptured relationships with their adolescents. To effectively engage in retrospective reflection, parents must recognize the hurts they suffered in their own parent–child relationship. It is important for them to identify the needs that were inadequately or inappropriately fulfilled, or totally unfulfilled. It is also important for parents to know what coping strategies they used—what worked well and what didn't. This process is ultimately designed to enhance parents' insight and understanding regarding the influences of their parent–child relationships on how they parent. For example, the parent who was never held or hugged as a child can now begin to see how this childhood behavior has influenced his or her own approach to parenting and how it might be connected to the disruption of community currently experienced by the adolescent.

Know the Center of Their Universe

We believe that it is never too late for a parent (or parents) to reverse old negative habits and interactions. Parents cannot actively promote the restoration of community if they are estranged from the world of their adolescent. If the adolescent is given lots of emotional and physical space to go adrift and keep his or her world totally isolated, there is little hope of restoring community. We believe that it is of paramount importance for parents to spend quality time with their adolescents and to know what constitutes the center of their universe. We certainly are aware of all the challenges that make this task so difficult. For example, the last thing that many adolescents at this stage want to do is to spend more time with their parents. Moreover, it is also common for parents to experience a comparable level of dread when it comes to spending more time with their adolescent, whom they often find to be painfully self-centered and obnoxious. In spite of these hurdles, it is imperative that parents spend quality time with their adolescents and know what is important to them. We are not suggesting that parents have to condone whatever constitutes the center of their adolescents' universe, but we do believe that it is important for them to be intimately familiar with it.

Demonstrate Vulnerability

We have made numerous references to vulnerability throughout this book. Obviously, we believe it a very important dimension of relationship development. Vulnerability paves the pathways to emotional connectedness. Our use of the term really refers to a process whereby parents (for our intended purpose here) have a willingness to openly express and address very sensitive emotions in the most delicate ways. In a practical sense, demonstrating vulnerability means that a parent (or parents) will engage with their adolescent on issues and topics that are highly sensitive, even discomforting, to approach. Demonstrating vulnerability is not just a matter of "what" is stated but also "how" it is stated. Thus, we believe, for example, that a parent who is worried or curious about his or her adolescents' sexual activity and addresses the issue with humor, indirect comments, or sarcasm would fail this task. Even though the *what* (topic) fits the bill, the *how* sends a dangerous message to the adolescent about vulnerability as well as the significance of the issue. When parents demonstrate vulnerability effectively, they are able to stay engaged in the most difficult interactions while also respectfully tolerating the adolescents' discomfort, rage, or pain. It is much easier for parents to make the shift from criticizing their adolescents to comforting them when they are comfortable with expressions of vulnerability. Share your experiences from your own childhood, including things you struggled with and things you may have done that you are not proud of now.

Take Personal Responsibility

This strategy is an outgrowth of the preceding one, and considerable vulnerability is required to execute it effectively. Parents who take personal responsibility have the ability to understand and acknowledge the ways in which they might have intentionally or unintentionally hurt their children. This means that the parents who put their newborn infant up for adoption would be able and willing to explain the circumstances to their 16-year-old daughter who spent 8 years locating them. Often it seems difficult for some parents, particularly those who feel blamed by their children, to take responsibility for their disruptive or hurtful behavior. When confronted with a hostile, blaming, and personally attacking offspring—especially one who has violated the law—most parents find it difficult to resist counterattacking or highlighting the adolescents' troubles. If parents really want to be effective in their efforts to repair relationships and restore community, taking personal responsibility in a vulnerable, nondefensive way is crucial.

It is important to note here that we do not view this as a one-time isolated technique. Parents don't simply take responsibility once or twice and adolescents magically begin to trust and form meaningful attachments to others. If anything, the most common initial response from most violent and aggressive youth is either disdain or hostility. The adolescents' response, however, should not deter parents from carrying out this task. If anything, the presence of such strong emotion from the adolescent should strengthen parents' resolve to take personal responsibility. In our therapy, we usually consider these "strong inappropriate" responses by adolescents as their effort to disconnect from more vulnerable emotions.

Listen Therapeutically

Listening therapeutically is really about listening to hear. It refers to a process in which parents are curious and seeking meaning rather than lecturing or offering unsolicited advice. It is the type of listening that facilitates a conversational tone and conveys to the speaker that "you are important to me and I am very interested in what you have to say—tell me more." Listening therapeutically also involves parents being proactive in encouraging adolescents to share all of their thoughts, feelings, and experiences while remaining open to and nonjudgmental about the things that are difficult to hear.

Integrate the VCR Approach into Everyday Life

We discussed the VCR approach in great detail in Chapter 7. We believe that it is critical for parents of violent and aggressive adolescents to use validation liberally. This is often necessary in order to counteract devaluation and begin to rebuild trust, safety, and security. Rather than incessantly challenging or criticizing adolescents, parents should use the VCR approach to achieve a greater balance among challenges, affirmations, and requests.

See the Good Contained in the Bad

Adolescents who do bad things often get defined by their misdeeds. Unfortunately, when they act violently or aggressively, the tendency to be labeled narrowly is exacerbated. When this happens it becomes very difficult for parents and others to notice any redeeming qualities, traits, or behaviors that the adolescent might possess. Repairing strained relationships and restoring community require parents to notice the good things that adolescents do and to take the time to acknowledge and praise these positive attributes. Some parents often believe that bad kids have to do something positively stellar before they should be praised, while other parents deliberately withhold praise because they are mistrustful of the adolescents' motives, which they usually characterize as attempts at manipulation.

Effectively Negotiate Different Agendas

Even under the best of circumstances, it is common for parents and adolescents to have divergent values, interests, and needs. *How these differences are resolved* is usually far more significant than the actual differences themselves. If domination, force, or manipulation is used, it can have long-lasting negative effects on the parent–adolescent relationship. In fact, these are the types of parent–driven interactions that trigger erosion of the primary community. On the

other hand, restoring community requires parents to effectively negotiate the different agendas that exist between them and their adolescents. A critical dimension of community involves negotiating different agendas so that everyone's perspectives and interests are taken
into consideration. It is important for parents to realize that they may
have to accept that their adolescents may want things for themselves
that are diametrically opposed to how they have been socialized. Our
use of the word "accept" here means to genuinely compromise and
embrace adolescents' positions without animosity, reprisal, or emotional cutoff. This in no way is intended to imply that we believe that
parents are compelled to agree with the differences.

Never Give Up

Charlie Levister, father of 16-year-old Danielle, stated rather elo-
quently what most parents of adolescents experience at some point as
he sat in my (KVH) office in a bewildered state: "I don't know what
my role is anymore . . . I don't seem to matter to her as much as I used
to—on a bad day I could actually feel 'used and abused.' I seem to be
good only for transportation when the better options don't pan out—
and, of course, money. Sometimes it's hard being with her, knowing
that I only serve a utilitarian purpose, as she glances at me through
the rear-view mirror." Mr. Levister was obviously hurting in response
to the unwelcomed shifts in his relationship with Danielle. He obviously longed for "the good ol' days" when he was the center of her life.
Back then, he felt loved, needed, and respected—all of which seem to
be a mere distant memory for him now. Mr. Levister is flirting with
the temptation of distancing himself from Danielle as a means of insu-
lating himself from the pains of letting go. Danielle's "rejection" of
him is more than he can stand, at the moment. We believe that what
Danielle and her father need most is for him to hang in there and not
to give up. Parents like Mr. Levister have to find ways to stay involved
with their adolescents—*especially* when they feel rejected. Parents who
can "weather the storm" and reject feeling rejected teach their adolescents valuable life lessons about trust building, unconditional love,
and the importance of relational connectedness.

Think Connection, Think Community

Thinking connection, thinking community is an important task
because it punctuates the significance of relatedness and relationships. When parents think connection, think community, they become

acutely aware of how central relationships are to our core as human beings. To repair disrupted relationships there must be a very strong emphasis on promoting connection. To reconnect with their disconnected and often disaffected adolescents, parents must be vigilant in their pursuit and support of connection. As therapists, we spend an extraordinary amount of time in therapy working tirelessly to help parents and adolescents to preserve the sanctity of their connection, even when both are unsure it's worth the effort. We believe this is in part what it means to think connection, think community. It means that we recognize that we are relational beings and that we live our lives in a relational context. In the world of violent and aggressive adolescents, this task means that a fed-up, severely disappointed parent will still give higher priority to his or her son's court date than to being present for an important business meeting. It shapes the behavior of the parent who decided that he or she will support the daughter's choice for a boyfriend even though he or she detests virtually everything about him. These are the types of easy decisions to difficult situations that parents can make when they are successful in thinking connection, thinking community.

As therapists, we have experienced substantial professional fallout in our effort to remain true to this task as a philosophical stance. Philosophically we believe that violent and aggressive adolescents who have some semblance of meaningful connections in their lives have a greater prognosis in therapy. We believe this to be the case even when the meaningful connection is not a healthy one, as in the case of gang membership. However, our premise is that gang membership, which we believe is the adolescent's effort to re-establish a primary community, requires some relationship skills. Gang membership requires loyalty, respect for hierarchy, rules, and boundaries, etc. Clinically, we believe it is important for us to support the gang-involved adolescent client's orientation toward relational connectedness while disavowing the gang activity. This has been an exceedingly difficult position to sell to parents and fellow colleagues alike. We hear repeatedly that it flirts too close to the line of supporting kids in gangs. Of course, from our perspective, nothing could be farther from the truth for us as therapists and as human beings. We do, on the other hand, stand guilty as charged if the claim is that we are thinking connection, thinking community.

It has been our experience that some parents are able to successfully implement these tasks while others find some or all of them very difficult to master. There are a multitude of reasons why these efforts can fail, ranging from philosophical differences among parents to a loss of optimism that anything can make a difference. Unfortunately, there are also situations where the disruptions in parent–teen relationships have been so severely damaging that healing and restoration require the supportive services of a trained professional, such as a family therapist. One of the first major tasks of the therapist is to facilitate parents' efforts to successfully implement the steps for repairing the relationships with their adolescents. Therapists can assume the role of coach and provide much-needed guidance and support to parents and adolescents. There are also a number of other more specific actions that therapists can take to help promote the restoration of community.

How Therapists Can Repair Parent–Adolescent Relationships

Therapists can use themselves to promote the restoration of primary community in the lives of adolescents in two basic ways.

1. The relationships therapists develop with their adolescent clients have great healing potential. Therefore, the first small step to restoring primary community involves the relationship that develops between therapist and client. In a sense, the therapist becomes a transferential parental object for the adolescent.
2. Therapists need to be doggedly determined about engaging as many family members as possible in the therapy process, especially parents. By incorporating parents into the therapy process, therapists have a much better chance of creating a safe, healing context that can ultimately focus on repairing strained relationships between parents and teens. Obviously, given the gravity of the strain, this process could take quite a bit of time and effort.

Adolescents who have strained relationships with their parents are usually very reluctant to have their parents included in the therapy process. Fear of criticism, disapproval, and rejection often makes it hard for them to entertain the idea of having their parents come to therapy. These fears are often intensified when adolescents feel a great deal of anger and bitterness toward their parents. Similarly, some parents may also be reticent to get involved in the therapy. They may be so frustrated and disillusioned with their adolescents that they can only contemplate giving up. Many parents appear disinterested and apathetic, which often is a response to feeling burned out and overwhelmed by the many struggles they have experienced with their adolescent. Other parents are so consumed with rage toward their adolescents that they push them away punitively. These parents are flooded with anger that drives them to distance themselves from their kids. On the occasions when these parents do interact with their adolescents, these exchanges almost always are characterized by bitterness and hostility.

Whatever the reasons underlying why it may be hard to get parents involved in their adolescents' therapy, their participation is vital. In fact, the more reticence there is, the more vital their involvement becomes. In cases where it is difficult to get parents involved in the therapy, there are several therapeutic stages and strategies we recommend that therapists follow to begin the restoration of primary community between parents and adolescents.

Stage 1: Positioning

The first stage consists of therapists positioning themselves. At the beginning of therapy, therapists must maneuver themselves in ways that are designed to connect with clients and gain access to the various parts of their clients' relational systems.

1. *Establishing a connection by exploring clients' meaning systems.* During the initial phase of therapy, therapists should strive to understand clients' meaning systems. Therapists should ask themselves, "How does this person make sense of the world and his or her place in it?" The conversation in this stage should be casual and relaxed. The major therapeutic goal at this stage is to get to know the adolescent sitting in front of them. Therapists should be actively piecing together the framework their client uses to make sense of the world, and the types of things that are important to him or her. The point of this, at least initially, is to explore what avenues will allow for the greatest possibility for a connection with each adolescent.

2. *Assessing the disruption to community in their clients' lives.* It is important for therapists to explore where the disruptions of community have occurred, because this will point to where the therapy will need to go in terms of the restoration of community. Once therapists have a basic understanding of where the disruptions occurred, they can begin to think critically and creatively about how to gain access to these other parts of their clients' lives. Therapists must begin to

formulate a plan for how to make contact with and engage these other parts of the system. For example, if there is a disruption in a client's school experience, the therapist needs to start thinking about how he or she can connect with the school to advocate on the client's behalf and ultimately restore community in terms of the client's relationship to school.

Stage 2: Making Contact

After therapists have "positioned" themselves with their clients (in terms of gaining insight into their meaning systems and access into different parts of their relational system), it's time to move to the next stage of the therapy, which consists of drawing the clients' parents into the therapy process. To accomplish this, we recommend the following.

1. *Encourage clients to try to get their parents to come in.* It is our belief that therapists should first prepare adolescents to make contact with their parents and ask them directly to come into therapy. This preparation should consist of helping adolescents explore how they will approach their parents and how they will respond to any number of potential responses. It is often helpful to role-play several different situations to give clients an opportunity to practice how they will interact with their parents under various circumstances. For clients who are particularly wary and fearful of approaching their parents, therapists can have them prepare either an audio- or videotape in which they make the request. Again, therapists should assist clients in preparing the tapes so that they represent an appropriate level of openness and vulnerability. The goal, above all, is to ensure that clients do not approach their parents in accusatory, angry, or otherwise negative ways. Our intent at this phase of the process is to begin disrupting old nonworking but well-established patterns that help to maintain distance and disconnection between adolescent and parent. This is why the advance, methodical preparation is necessary. Our belief is that if the parent and the adolescent are left to their own devices at this point the old nonworking patterns will prevail.

2. *Contact parents directly when adolescents don't succeed in getting their parents to come in.* If adolescents' efforts to get their parents to come to therapy fail, the next step is for therapists to contact parents directly. When therapists call, it is important that they assume a negotiating stance and not resort to strong-arm tactics. Therapists should

make it clear that they are soliciting parents' input and asking them to serve as consultants in the therapy. For example, therapists could say, "You know your child better than I do, and I think I could really benefit from your assistance in my work with him." It also is helpful for therapists to negotiate in advance the number of sessions that parents will attend—for example, "If you would agree to come to two sessions with your son, this would be very helpful." Therapists might also create a caveat that if, at the conclusion of the two sessions, the parents want to attend additional sessions, it could be renegotiated at that time.

Stage 3: Preparation

Once parents have agreed to attend, the next stage involves preparation. We seldom embark on a conjoint session between estranged parents and adolescents without extensive preparatory sessions. We consider this phase of our work the "reconstructive." The work during this stage is delicate but necessary. We spend quite a bit of time with the adolescents and the parents separately. Our goal is to get a better idea of what each perceives as opportunities and obstacles. We also use this time to adequately prepare them for what the process will invariably involve and to anticipate what some of the "speed bumps" along the way might be. In essence, our goal is to prepare them for major "surgery." It has been our experience that the conjoint sessions are much more productive when the parents and adolescents have been appropriately prepped beforehand.

Prepping Adolescents. Preparing adolescents is critical, because one can never predict how a parent will respond in a session, and if they respond harshly, the adolescent must be prepared. We learned this the hard way during a session we once conducted with a 16-year-old girl and her stepmother. The stepdaughter was devastated after her stepmother attacked her during the session. The stepdaughter not only felt angry with and hurt by her stepmother, but she also felt betrayed by us as her therapists who had failed to prepare and protect her.

Sometimes it is helpful to imagine different ways the sessions might go and to use guided imagery techniques to help clients explore how they will feel and respond to the different scenarios. It is especially useful to prepare adolescents for the worst—that is, being rejected by their parents. To help prepare adolescents for this possibility, we recommend using metaphors. In our work we select a metaphor that has relevance to the adolescent we're working with, and we use it to give him or her a way of thinking about the worst possible scenario in images that make it seem tolerable rather than devastating. For example, in our therapy with a 15-year-old male, Steve, we drew on his deep love and talent for basketball. To prepare him for the possibility of rejection in the session with his mother, we said to him:

> "It's like bringing a star player into a team during the midseason. He's obviously a great player, but because he's coming into a new situation without the benefit of the preseason time to develop a rhythm with his new team, he may actually start out by playing worse. He and the team may not seem like a good fit. But they just need some time together to work it out. It's not about either of them being inadequate—it doesn't mean they won't develop a great chemistry eventually—it's just going to take a while, especially since they started out under such challenging conditions."

The point is to prepare adolescents by using their existing meaning systems in a metaphorical way. Metaphors can be powerful vehicles for cognitive and emotional transformation. In the case of Steve, a boy who loved basketball, we used basketball as a metaphor for discussing his mother's participation in therapy. It was our hope that Steve would transfer his thoughts and feelings about basketball to his relationship with his mother. Ideally, this transference was intended to provide Steve with a meaningful way of relating to his experience with his mother.

To conclude the preparatory work with adolescents, therapists should have adolescents identify one or two things they would need to have happen in the conjoint sessions to feel some sense of hopefulness. It should be something small and achievable. If it's something too lofty, the session will only be a set-up for disappointment, so therapists should guide adolescents in focusing upon small, "bite-size" pieces of hope.

Prepping Parents. In addition to preparing adolescents, it also is important to prepare their parents. Parents should be invited to attend a presession during which they meet alone with the therapist. During the presession therapists work to give the parents a different way of thinking about their adolescents. Therapists might use some piece of an adolescent's story or words to try to promote a different type of connection between the parent and adolescent. For example, when

Steve's mother came in for her presession, we mentioned to her that Steve still remembers the time she came to his basketball game when he was 8. In a sense, we serve as Steve's voice, conveying parts of his story to his mother in an effort to forge a positive connection between the two. By telling Steve's mother that he still remembers her visiting his game, we were giving her something hopeful to hang on to in their relationship. We also wanted to give his mother an empathic way of thinking about Steve (i.e., as a vulnerable little boy).

It also is important for therapists to use the presession as a forum for reporting some good news to parents about their adolescents. Again, we want to begin from a position of hopefulness, so we infuse something positive about an adolescent's progress as a way of encouraging the parents to think about the adolescent in a hopeful way.

Toward the end of the presession the therapists should ask parents to identify one or two things they would like to see happen in the conjoint session to feel more hopeful about their relationship with their adolescent.

Stage 4: The Conjoint Sessions

The next stage of the therapy involves the conjoint sessions with parents and adolescents. During these sessions therapists should strive for small but significant steps toward repairing the relationship. The therapist should function as a negotiator who is trying to bring together parents and adolescents in the hope of forging and/or reviving a fragile connection. This is accomplished by trying to open up new ways for each to think about the other. If both parties can see the other in a more empathic and hopeful light, it will allow both parties to take small but significant steps toward each other. In our work we also use this time to outline and reinforce the important tasks that we believe parents have to be willing to engage in, in the interest of repairing the injury to their relationship with their child.

A Word about Other Family Members

Therapists can also help restore primary community in the lives of adolescents by nurturing relationships between adolescents and other family members. Therapists should draw as many people into the therapy process as possible—siblings, grandparents, aunts, uncles, and cousins—anyone who is a part of an adolescent's relational sphere.

It also is important to consider the role that peers often play in terms of primary community in the lives of adolescents. The more disrupted families become, the more teens tend to rely on their peer groups as surrogate families—or, as therapist Ron Taffel (2001) puts it, as their "Second Family." Like families, peer groups become primary locations where adolescents derive a sense of safety, nurturance, acceptance, socialization, and sense of connectedness. Especially for teens who have family problems, who feel like outcasts at school, or who have suffered from various kinds of culturally based bigotry and intolerance, a few good friends often become the salve adolescents reach for to soothe their pain. Hence, efforts to promote the restoration of community in the lives of adolescents should draw heavily on the resource that is reflected in peer relationships. Consequently, in situations where friends have close, significant bonds with teenaged clients, we believe it is important to include them in the therapy process as well (see Laszloffy, 2000 for more on how to conduct peer group therapy).

How Other Concerned Adults Can Repair Parent–Adolescent Relationships

Teachers and other concerned adults (e.g., clergy, coaches, juvenile probation officers) may be limited in their capacity to promote the restoration of community at the primary level. It is much harder for those who are not family members or therapists (whose job is to deal directly with family relationships) to promote the restoration of community at the primary level. Nonetheless, in many cases the best one can do is to reach out to develop (and sustain) a healthy, healing primary relationship with an adolescent. By establishing a relationship with a teen that offers guidance, boundaries, caring, and love, adults who are not family and not therapists can cultivate ties with teens that foster a sense of community at the primary level.

EXTENDED COMMUNITY

Indicators of Disruptions to Community at the Extended Level

Before the restoration of community at the extended level can be promoted among adolescents, it is first necessary to accurately identify where specific disruptions exist. Sometimes disruptions of community at the extended level involve broad events or conditions that are greater than a single person. For example, each of the schools across the nation where shootings have occurred is an example of an extended community that has endured massive disruptions. The victims of those shootings were not limited to the children and adults who sustained physical injuries. All of the students in the school, the staff, their families, and the town residents were ravaged by the attacks. All of the factors that define community were assaulted with these acts of violence. The sense of trust, safety, and closeness within these communities was severely assaulted by the adolescent shooters who turned to egregious acts of violence targeting their extended community.

When economically impoverished neighborhoods are ravaged by drugs and crime, it severely undermines one's sense of community. It has never been surprising to us to hear so many young people refer to where they live as "the hood." It almost appears as if they know intuitively what is missing from this characterization: one's neighbor. We believe of course that one's "neighbor" is the basis for connection— without it, there is only the hood. In so many of these locations, young people are deprived of opportunities to develop a positive sense of kinship with the area that exists just beyond their front door. The types of caring good-neighbor experiences that are characteristic of strong, healthy neighborhoods is denied to children who grow up in crime-infested areas plagued by danger and distrust.

Being able to identify how individual adolescents are affected by disruptions to their extended communities is important. Some try to compensate by getting involved in "negative communities." For many teens, the "negative" community they find in gangs is preferable to no community at all. Kids who turn to gangs are reaching out desperately for a sense of community wherever they can find it. When we meet with kids who are involved with gangs, it is almost always the case that these are kids who don't feel connected anywhere else in their lives. These are kids who feel utterly alienated from the world around them. They feel rejected, lost, and alone. To fulfill their desperate longing for a sense of community many adolescents turn to gangs as the only place where they can find meaningful ties with others. As reported to us by Troy, a teenaged boy who was in a gang: "My family doesn't know if I'm alive, and they don't care. But it goes both ways. I don't care about them either. I care about my G's [fellow gang members], though. We look out for each other. My G's are my family." Troy clearly had experienced the disruption of his primary community, and he had counteracted this loss by joining a gang. His G's and the gang provided him with the family he had been missing.

We interpret gang involvement as a rather obvious indicator of the disruption of community at the extended (and often primary) level. Adolescents in gangs often say they joined because they needed protection against other adolescents or gangs. The fact that young people feel the need to turn to gangs for safety speaks to the failure of their families, schools, and neighborhoods to provide the safety to which all children are entitled. All children have an inherent right to walk down a street without feeling fear. When youth are robbed of this basic freedom, it implies that the "legitimate" communities in their lives have shirked their responsibility to ensure this freedom.

In some instances, disruptions to an adolescent's community at the extended level can be unique to that individual. Overall, the school, neighborhood, and other extended communities that adolescents are members of may appear stable, cohesive, and safe. Yet, at the same time, individual adolescents may have personal experiences that result in a sense of disruption at the extended level of community. Adolescents who are rebuffed by other adolescents and treated as outcasts often experience disruptions at the extended level. These adolescents suffer from intense social isolation and ostracism, which is a very strong indicator of a sense of disruption at this level for those individuals. When adolescents are loners or outcasts who seem only loosely connected to others and spend most of their time alone, this should be treated as a red flag.

It is important that adults make critical distinctions between kids who genuinely prefer spending time alone, versus those who are alone in response to peer rejection. One of us (TAL) was definitely one of those kids who preferred to be alone as a child. I thought there was nothing more stimulating than working in my room on any number of art projects that I loved to dream up. Creative expression was my passion, and I worked most joyfully when I had blocks of time alone to immerse myself in my creations. The difference between this type of aloneness and the type of behavior we find worrisome depends on how the youth perceives his or her isolation. In my case, I chose to spend a lot of time alone because I genuinely enjoyed time by myself. It wasn't a response to feeling rejected by other kids. In fact, I had many friends who complained that I wasn't more sociable. They wanted me to spend more time with them than I did. I also was heavily involved in studying ballet and went every day after school for lessons. Through this activity I became a member of a rich social network that provided a dramatic contrast to the many hours I spent alone in my room painting and drawing.

The type of loner behavior that we believe warrants concern involves adolescents who spend large chunks of time alone because they feel rejected by other kids. Sometimes this can be hard to assess because teens often try to protect themselves against the pain of rejection by denying that they have been rejected (e.g., a common sentiment is "They didn't reject me—I rejected them because I wouldn't want to be friends with those kids if they were the last kids on earth"). To "save face," they commonly say things that are designed to give the impression that their isolation is a choice—their preferred choice. But once subjected to closer scrutiny, it is possible to see the difference between those adolescents who genuinely feel okay about their aloneness versus those who are merely projecting a false sense of being okay as a way of avoiding disrespect.

Again we refer to Eric Harris and Dylan Klebold. Here were two boys that suffered from extreme isolation and peer rejection. Both boys had been taunted at school by other kids who called them weirdos and rejects. In response to peer rejection, Eric and Dylan spent a lot of time together tucked away isolated from other people. But the difference between the creative projects they were working on in their rooms and the ones I worked on in my room when I was their age was that between night and day. Eric and Dylan perceived themselves as having been scorned by other kids. No matter how they might have postured in an effort to suggest their aloneness was a preferred and positive choice, in reality both boys were alone because they had been snubbed by other adolescents. This was made clear in their letters and video diaries, where they acknowledged the social ostracism they had suffered and expressed rage and bitterness in response to this.

Sometimes adolescents form "outcast clubs," or gangs, in response to social rejection. Eric and Dylan were members of a group called the "trenchcoat Mafia," which was formed when individual teens who felt socially scorned came together and bonded on the basis of their status as "rejects." Or as one 13-year-old boy who was a member of a street gang once told us, "My G's are the only real friends I ever had. Before them, I basically didn't have any friends. Now I got friends—and ones I know I can count on for anything." Adults need to have an internal radar system that alerts them to the quality of adolescents' social status and their relationships with other kids. Even among adolescents who claim to not care what others think of them, social approval is one of the most powerful organizing principles during this stage of life. So, it becomes crucial to notice how many friends an adolescent has and how young people spend their free time and with whom. Adults need to be tuned into the types of social networks kids are involved in, and they have to look for signs of peer rejection and ostracism (e.g., hyperbolic pronouncements about not needing friends or caring what anyone else thinks). Whether in our respective roles as parents, therapists, teachers, coaches, or clergy, we need to be tuned into the broader networks with which adolescents are involved. It is important for each of us to know what's happening with adolescents in school, who their friends are, where they hang out, what's happening in the neighborhoods where they live, and what types of activities and organizations they are involved in. This type of awareness is critical to being able to see and understand how teens might be struggling with disruptions of community at the extended level.

How Parents Can Promote Restoration of Community at the Extended Level

There are several ways that parents can assume an active role in helping to promote the restoration of community at the extended level. When parents are aware of a disruption within an entire community, they should use whatever power they have to address the disruption. For example, a group of concerned parents in a crime-infested urban housing project formed a caring community coalition that restored a sense community to their neighborhood. They formed a neighborhood "cleanup" project that focused on banishing the criminal elements that were sucking the life out of their community and their children's future.

Parents also need to use their radar to identify any signs that their teens might be suffering from the pain of social rejection and alienation. They need to notice the friends their adolescents have (or, just as importantly, do *not* have). Parents need to be close observers of their children's lives. If they notice that their kids spend a lot of time alone, they need to explore the reasons for this. They also need to be curious about the types of activities their kids are involved in and the kinds of things that spark their interest and enthusiasm. If parents discover that their adolescents are struggling with peer rejection, talking with them and finding ways to send caring, supportive messages becomes extremely important.

If parents find out that their adolescents are involved in "negative social groups," it is important to first talk with them about why these groups are important to them. They should ask questions like "What do you like about this group of friends?" They should employ the techniques of the VCR approach as a vehicle for ultimately helping their adolescents transfer their loyalty from peers who may be a bad influence to ones that may be more positive. This means that parents also must assume an active role in creating avenues that will allow their adolescents to gain access to more positive peer networks. For example, a father could start coaching a softball team and encourage his daughter to join the team. A mother with a special skill, like photography, could teach a course for teens at the local community center and get her son involved. If a parent is connected to a youth counselor, priest, or rabbi who is especially "hip" and talented with kids, she might ask that person to reach out to her adolescent as a way of getting him or her connected with an adult who could open the door to a new community of peers.

How Therapists Can Promote Restoration of Community at the Extended Level

A critical part of the work that therapists do involves repairing relationships that exist on multiple levels simultaneously. In addition to focusing on the family system, therapists also must keep one eye focused on other social systems as well. Hence, it is important to attend to an adolescent's relationships with the members of their neighborhoods, their schools, religious organizations, and other clubs, agencies, teams, and groups that teens are involved with. For example, in the case of our 16-year-old client Steve, not only did we focus on reconnecting mother and son, but we also contacted Steve's teachers and his basketball coach. Since he was at risk of being kicked off the team and expelled from school for his drug use and suspected violent behavior, we intervened on his behalf. We got together with his teachers and coach and explained that Steve was at a critical place in his life—he was teetering on the line and could go either way. We believed that with support from the school it wasn't too late for him. We asked if they could give Steve another chance—but this time with all of us uniting to help him together.

In our sessions with Steve we knew that his suspension from the team was a major disruption of his sense of community at the extended level. We encouraged him to contact a few of the guys to arrange a time when they would get together routinely to work out. Even though he was suspended from the team, we wanted him to try to retain his connections with his teammates.

How Teachers Can Promote Restoration of Community at the Extended Level

Teachers work in one of the most important extended communities that adolescents are involved in, namely, schools. Therefore, teachers can and should play an instrumental role in promoting the restoration of community at this level. We also believe that teachers should focus their attention on promoting a strong, inclusive, positive sense of community both in their individual classrooms and within the school at large.

1. *Use teaching strategies that emphasize community and cooperation.* Whatever approach to education a teacher has, it is important to simultaneously focus on how classrooms can become places where adolescents learn to think about themselves as members of a whole that is greater than their individual selves. Classrooms should become places where kids learn to think about what it means to share resources, to help each other solve problems, and to communicate their own thoughts and feelings while being respectful of others. One very simple way of creating a context that supports a sense of community is by arranging desks and chairs in a semicircle so that students are able to look around the room and see each other. We encourage teachers to ask students to make sure that they can see the eyes of every other student in the classroom. Teachers can also convert larger classrooms into smaller learning communities by arranging desks in clusters that foster more direct, personal interactions between students.

A useful way of building community in classrooms is by assigning small group or class projects that require students to work as a team to achieve an overarching goal. For example, an English teacher we spoke with had her class work together to stage a dramatic performance of a play that they had read earlier in the year. The students were entirely responsible for the production including the management of the marginal budget she allocated to them. They were evaluated not only on the product they presented, but on how well they managed to work together as a collective, to negotiate conflicts as they arose, and to employ creative strategies to maneuver around obstacles.

Similarly, we have spoken with several science teachers who described using some variation on the concept of having their classes work collectively to devise and implement environmentally friendly projects incorporating what they are learning in class. Exercises like these achieve the dual objectives of having students apply class concepts in practical situations while simultaneously challenging them to work together for the common good.

One teacher we met proudly shared with us that she was familiar with the work of Virginia Satir, a well-known family therapist who developed humanistic, experientially-based exercises to teach families how to communicate effectively, build self-esteem, and foster healthy interpersonal relationships. This teacher excitedly shared with us how at the midpoint of the school year she led each of her classes through one of Satir's exercises. She said that she did this to teach essential life skills and to build community. For example, the Family Sculpture is an exercise where one family member creates a human sculpture with the other members of the family. The sculpture that is created reflects how this person sees the family and her or his position/role in that family. After the sculpture is completed the therapist processes with the members of the family how it felt to be in this sculpture and what they were able to understand about how the sculptor perceives them and the family overall.

While this exercise is targeted at families, this teacher effectively applied it with her classes, explaining that each class is like a family group. She was most enthusiastic about the ways in which this simple exercise and others like it helped her students to appreciate their interrelatedness and to consider things like how others perceive them, how they perceive others, how they feel about being a part of the class community, and how communication occurs on multiple levels, verbally and non-verbally, and involves thoughts, feelings, and behaviors. According to this teacher, the spirit of cooperation and the quality of communication always improved after she engaged her classes in an exercise like the Family Sculpture. While some teachers might feel hesitant about utilizing activities of this nature, we recommend reading Satir's book *Peoplemaking* to gain an understanding of her philosophy and to survey the particular exercises she presents.

2. *Notice and intervene when adolescents taunt and make fun of other kids.* Teachers have a critical responsibility with respect to encouraging pro-social development and positive relationship skills, which includes redirecting behaviors that consist of belittling and

shaming other kids. While it is common for kids to pick on each other, sometimes in very cruel ways, it is of particular concern when one or a group of teenagers singles another teenager out and repeatedly antagonizes, taunts, or harasses that individual, particularly where there is an unequal power between the aggressor(s) and the victim. Otherwise known as bullying behavior, this phenomenon has grown increasingly common in schools, and the devastation it can have on those who are targeted is serious.

Because bullying so often occurs in schools, teachers are on the frontlines and have a great responsibility to recognize the signs and symptoms of bullying and to know how to combat it effectively. In a general way we offer the following recommendations for how teachers can establish classroom environments that facilitate identifying and positively addressing bullying behaviors:

1. Develop class rules that discourage bullying behaviors;
2. Clarify what the consequences will be for bullying behaviors and follow through on implementing these in a consistent manner as necessary;
3. Affirm displays of pro-social behavior;
4. Actively promote and affirm the notion that diversity is valued and differences are okay;
5. Teach students how to negotiate and resolve conflicts using healthy communication skills;
6. Hold regular discussion groups and/or have students write compositions that address topics that are germane to issues that they struggle with on a day-to-day basis; for example, "Outcasts," "Respect and Disrespect," and "What makes someone cool?"

It is also important for school administrators to support policies and procedures for identifying and dealing with bullying behaviors, including providing staff with in-service trainings to educate them about the causes and consequences of bullying and to provide recommendations for how they can address it. We will not say more on this matter because it is beyond the scope of this book to discuss bullying and how to counteract it in schools, but there are several excellent resources we recommend including *Bullying at School: What We Know and What We Can Do (Understanding Children's Worlds)* by Dan Olweus; *And Words Can Hurt Forever: How to Protect Adolescents from Bullying, Harassment, and Emotional Violence* by James Garabino and Ellen Delara;

Bullying in Schools: Causes, Preventions, and Interventions by Anne Garrett; and *Respectful Schools: How Educators and Students Can Conquer Hate and Harassment* by Steve Wessler and William Preble.

How Other Adults Can Promote Restoration of Community at the Extended Level

Other concerned adults can take a proactive role in promoting the restoration of community at the extended level. For example, an athletic coach might commit himself to creating a sense of community among the members of his team. A pastor could decide to foster community within a Sunday school class or could form a youth group for kids within the congregation. A committed adult might found a youth club devoted to organizing positive initiatives within her neighborhood, like a neighborhood "cleanup," a tree-planting project, or a recycling initiative. An adult could decide to organize and coach a neighborhood baseball league with the broader goal of using the team as a forum for creating community among the adolescents who live in the area. A staff person at a local community center could establish a Tough Talk group for teens where they could come together to rap with one another about the struggles in their lives. The point in each of these scenarios is for a dedicated adult to use his or her talents and vision to bring together a group of adolescents and to create an experience that will blossom into "community."

It may be difficult initially to establish something that is truly creative. The kids themselves may demonstrate little interest in getting involved in certain types of groups. But we have seen what is possible when an adult is *determined*. Eventually kids connect with the passion that a strong leader ignites in others. It takes time, but where there is conviction, things eventually take off.

CULTURAL COMMUNITY

Indicators of Disruptions of Community at the Cultural Level

The best way to identify disruptions of cultural community is by talking with teens directly about these issues. When we conduct group work with adolescents, we are always amazed at how hungry they are to discuss issues pertaining to culture and diversity. Perhaps because adolescence is a time of identity exploration, most teens are obsessed with questions that focus on who they are and how they fit in with the surrounding world. Questions about diversity are a natural extension of their search to define themselves and their place in the world.

Our efforts to determine disruption in the cultural community are usually devoted to paying close attention to the views that adolescents hold about themselves in terms of their unique racial, gender, class, religious, and sexual orientation identities. It is instructive to know what types of experiences adolescents have had in terms of these parts of their identity. For example, in our therapy with a 17-year-old girl named Audrey who was severely depressed, we expanded our conversation with her to include a consideration of gender issues. We did this by asking her, "How often do you think of yourself as a girl? What's it like to be a girl in this society? If you could choose between being a boy or a girl, which would you choose and why? What do you like about yourself as a person? What would you change about yourself if you could?" These types of questions invited Audrey to explore her gender identity. As we had expected, Audrey thought a lot about what it meant to be a girl. In fact, she told us that she often thought it was too hard being a girl because it meant she had to be beautiful, with a tiny waist and slim thighs. According to Audrey, her thighs were too fat, her nose too big, and her breasts too small. She was jealous of girls who were more beautiful, and she felt rejected by boys and by girls who were beautiful. Her insecurities about her beauty and her struggles to become a "successful girl" played a key role in the depression. This conversation allowed us to see how, at the cultural level, Audrey did not have a strong, positive sense of herself in terms of gender. As a girl, she was tortured by feelings of self-doubt, insecurity, and alienation.

Adolescents who suffer from disruption of community at the cultural level fall broadly into one of two categories. The first consists of adolescents who experience some form of prejudice, discrimination, and societal devaluation on the basis of their membership in a socioculturally oppressed cultural community. For adolescents who belong to socioculturally oppressed groups (e.g., poor kids, kids of color, gay and lesbian youth), the quest for a strong sense of cultural community is partly tied to feeling targeted and devalued on the basis of their race, class, sexual orientation, religion, or gender. Audrey is such an example. In terms of her gender she felt extremely devalued. Timothy Ryan is an example of an adolescent who struggled deeply with feeling "less than" on the basis of his working-class background, while Daquon Jackson was a teen who has been mistreated as an African American. For Carmen Brody, her sense of cultural community had been disrupted in several ways. She suffered painfully from repeated experiences where she had been treated poorly as a person of color, as a female, and because of her Spanish accent.

Even adolescents who have membership in socially privileged groups can struggle with a sense of disruption in terms of cultural community. For example, the trend among middle-class white youth to adopt the dress, vernacular, and music of urban youth of color stems from a throbbing desire to feel a sense of cultural community. WASP adolescents often tell us they wish they were kids of color because they envy the cultural unity they perceive among African American and Latino youth. As one girl told us:

"All the black and Hispanic kids seem to have this strong connection because of their ethnicity. It makes me jealous because, as a white person, I don't feel that type of ethnic bond. And then when the black kids wear those tee-shirts that say 'It's a black thing, you wouldn't understand,' that really makes me mad. It's true I don't understand, but I want to. I feel excluded. And I don't have a group of my own to bond with. White people don't have the same cultural thing that unites us the way the black and Hispanic kids do."

This girl's remarks, while overlooking the invisible bonding that does in fact exist among whites, is describing the sense of alienation she personally feels in terms of her cultural community. We have seen other examples of this in our clinical practice. In the last several years, I (KVH) have received numerous self-referrals from white families where the request is for me to provide help to an adolescent who "acts too black." These parents are usually quite distressed that their adolescent's behavior falls outside of the social or cultural norms established by the family. However, for the adolescents, they all say virtually the same thing: "That this is not about trying to be black or anything . . . It's what I like and what I relate to . . . It's about being a part of the hip hop thing." Many have suggested that they either don't feel comfortable or relate to being white. Interestingly, this phenomenon is not limited to race; we see a number of poor adolescents who think of themselves as rich and rich kids who think of themselves as poor. Behaviors of this variety are usually strong indicators of disruption of community at the cultural level.

Promoting the Restoration of Community at the Cultural Level

For those of us committed to addressing the disruption of community at the cultural level, we can do so in two ways. The first consists of helping adolescents feel pride and confidence about the different dimensions of their (cultural) identities (e.g., as "Puerto Rican," "white," "African American," "male," "female," "gay," "Jewish," "straight," "Mormon," and so forth), especially when they might be devalued by the broader society.

During our therapy with Steve, we asked him directly about his experiences as an African American male within a race-conscious society, particularly growing up in a predominantly white neighborhood and attending an all-white school. It took him very little time before he began recalling a seemingly endless number of experiences where he felt hurt or singled out as an African American. "None of my teachers at school are black except for Mrs. Washington. It would be nice—I am not going to lie—if there were a few more black teachers. It's kinda tough, you know . . . not having people who look like you there to support you or teach you the way. I have some cool white teachers . . . They try . . . but I don't think it's the same. Just like there are some things that only your Pops can teach you as a dude, there are some things that only someone who looks like you can pass on. Yeah, it bothers me sometimes."

As a way of trying to lend support to Steve's feelings and assist him in connecting with his identity as a black male, one of the things we did was to recommend several books to him; *The Autobiography of Malcolm X, Native Son* (by Richard Wright), and *Makes Me Wanna Holler* (by Nathan McCall). These books provided Steve with examples of acclaimed black men who had written about similar struggles and how they had dealt with them. He read all three books in 2 weeks and was so inspired he wanted to write his own story as a result. By recommending these books to Steve, we were providing him with a map for how he could begin to establish a sense of connection in terms of his cultural identity. This was a first step in promoting the restoration of community at the cultural level in Steve's life.

Our work with Steve was also a reminder of why it is important for those of us who work with violent and aggressive youth to assume the role of cultural translator. We recognized with Steve (as is the case with so many of the other adolescents with whom we work) that a huge piece of what he needed from us was some way to better understand the complexity of his condition as an African American male.

There were questions, concerns, and experiences that he had that were begging for acknowledgment, conversation, and deconstruction. All of these issues were connected to the cultural community and under most circumstances would be beyond the purview of the more traditional clinical approaches to working with troubled youth. For example, how was Steve to understand why he was constantly ridiculed for "talking white," or teased for going to a "white school," or constantly overlooked by the cashier at a sandwich shop near school at the same time he was closely monitored and followed while in the store? It was painfully clear to us that these were big areas of concern for Steve. There was a painful disconnect between how he saw himself and how he was perceived by others. In some ways, he was far too white for his black friends, too noticeably black for store officials while shopping, and invisible when at the cashier's station in the presence of other white patrons. Over time, and perhaps with age, Steve will make sense out of the nonsense, provided he does not inappropriately explode first. But for adolescents like Steve, these are very complex issues to sort through, especially in isolation without the help of someone conversant with the nuances of the cultural community.

A second way of addressing the disruption of community at the cultural level is by each of us taking an active role in confronting the unjust social conditions that contribute to racial, gender, class, sexual orientation, and religious oppression. Challenging even the smallest expressions of oppression is important, whether it's an expression that comes from within us or from the surrounding environment. The goal is to make the world a safer place for all people and a place where differences of all types can be respected and allowed to flourish, free from denigration or attack.

Quan was a 16-year-old Asian American who was referred to us by his school guidance counselor. He had written several essays with strong undertones of violence that had his teachers and school officials worried. Quan told us that he felt like a misfit in school. "I'm a freak," he said. We asked him to describe to us the ways in which he felt like a freak. At first he was vague: "I just don't fit in." But we persevered and continued to pursue specifics about how he felt like he didn't fit in. The first things he said seemed calculated and guarded: "I'm so quiet, not rowdy like the other boys. I like to study a lot. I hate sports."

"Do you have any friends at all? Have you dated anyone?"

"I don't really have too many friends. I sometimes hang out with the other Asian kids, but mostly I keep to myself. As for dating, I don't want to date anyone. That's another way that I'm a freak."

We didn't really think that Quan had no interest in dating. We suspected that he was gay and probably did not feel the freedom or safety to date whom he wanted to. When we shared our hypothesis with him, he denied it vehemently but uncomfortably. He stared at us for a moment and then began to cry. He eventually acknowledged that he was gay and said it was a huge relief to finally tell someone. His fear of rejection and punishment had kept him in the closet until now.

After Quan came out as a gay male, for the first time in his life he was able to discuss his true feelings. He spoke of his fear and shame, and his frustration and loneliness. In fact, many of the violent essays that Quan had written were symbolic of fantasies that he perpetually had about striking back at "his persecutors," as he called them. While it was therapeutic for Quan to express these feelings, the restoration of his sense of cultural community required that we do more than just talk with him. One of the things we did was help Quan get connected with other gay youth as a way of establishing a sense of cultural community as a young gay male. This was the first opportunity he had ever had to talk with other kids like himself.

With Quan's permission, we also contacted his guidance counselor and spoke with her about heterosexism and homophobia within the school. Based on things that Quan had shared with us, we were concerned about the number of flagrant and unchallenged expressions of homophobia in his school that made it an unsafe and unsupportive environment for gay, lesbian, and bisexual youth. Fortunately, Quan's guidance counselor was very responsive to the issues we raised. She agreed to spearhead the introduction of several progay initiatives within the school. We directed her to several organizations that specifically focus on making schools safe communities for youth of all sexual orientations. These types of actions were critical in helping to promote a strong, positive cultural community in terms of sexual orientation, not only for Quan but also for all of the gay, lesbian, and bisexual teens in his school.

CARMEN'S STORY: A CASE EXAMPLE OF PROMOTING THE RESTORATION OF COMMUNITY

In Carmen's case, the relationship between all three levels of community was interconnected, which meant we did not address each level of community discretely or sequentially. Our work occurred in a much more overlapping and zigzagging fashion. However, we did begin at the primary level, where the relationship between Carmen and her parents needed to be strengthened. We knew she loved her parents, yet she did not feel the trust to share her pain with them. And, while the Brodys loved their daughter, despite their desire to support her, they did not see or understand how much loneliness and hurt she carried inside. We needed to find ways to build greater safety and openness between Carmen and her parents. Doing so would open the door to addressing her disruptions of community in terms of the death of her birth parents, her separation from the village of her childhood and her country of origin, and her alienation at school, which was tied to her disrupted cultural identity as a girl of color within a predominantly white environment.

During our fourth session with Carmen we began the work of preparing her for conjoint therapy with her parents. We had her consider what things she secretly wished she could tell them but was always afraid to. We explored what kept her silent and what would have to happen to open her up with them. We walked her through worst-case scenarios regarding how her parents might respond if she were to share some of what she had been holding inside all these years.

While we were preparing Carmen, we began to meet alone with her parents to begin preparing them as well for our conjoint sessions. We explored with them how much they knew of Carmen's history before they adopted her. How did they learn what they knew? How often did they speak with Carmen about all of this? What did they say to her? What overt or covert rules had shaped Carmen's initiation and acceptance into their family? What private fears or concerns did they have when they first adopted Carmen, and how did they deal with these? What private worries did they have about her now, and how did they cope with these? How did they negotiate their racial, cultural, religious, and class differences? We also asked them to consider: What would be the worst thing they could find out about Carmen and their relationship with her? Then we had them walk through what they would do if these fears ever came to fruition. Through these types of questions we were setting a stage for the Brodys to begin thinking about what might be going on with Carmen, and we were preparing them for an open, truth-telling conversation.

During the conjoint session, we began by observing that this family's members loved one another so much that they were all trying to protect one another by not talking about painful things. But ironically, in their efforts to protect one another, the silences between them were hurting all of them. We started with the Brodys and had them, as the parents, take the first risk. Because they had been prepped, they were ready to open things up and began by sharing the joy and the worries they had when they first adopted Carmen. She was precious to them from the first day, and they wanted to protect her—to spare her pain. They assumed the best way to do this was to leave the past in the past and to give Carmen a new start with them.

She cried when she heard this. We pursued why she was crying. She said she was so grateful to them because they did give her a new start and a wonderful life.

"But then why are you so unhappy?" Carmen's mother asked.

Carmen took the next risk by saying that she wanted her life with them to work as much as they did. She never wanted to burden them with her struggles. She wanted to be the perfect daughter. Mrs. Brody broke down in tears.

"You are the perfect daughter just the way you are. Nothing you could tell us would change that."

Mrs. Brody was giving Carmen permission to say more. With some coaching Carmen took a few more steps and told her parents that she knew they loved her, but the truth was that she still felt like an outsider in the family.

"I'm not like the rest of you, and I never will be—no matter how hard I try."

"But we don't want you to be anyone but yourself," Mr. Brody replied.

With some coaxing Carmen confessed she did not believe this entirely. She reminded her parents of a time when she was 8 and wanted to play along in a game that some other kids were playing. "This girl told me to go play with the other niggers. I had only been here a few months when that happened, so I'd never heard that word before, but I knew it was bad. Mom, when I asked you about that word I still remember you telling me it was a bad word to call black people, but I shouldn't worry because I wasn't black. You told me you were my mother and you weren't black and neither was I. That's when I knew that I had to be white."

Her parents looked stunned, but there was light we could see in their eyes. Something was becoming clear to them. Carmen went on to remind them how they never talked about Peru or the fact that her family was murdered, or that they and she were poor rural people of color. Carmen then started to cry again and said, "I feel so confused. I feel like who I am is bad, which is why we can never talk about it. But I also know you love me, and I am afraid I'm hurting you now."

Carmen's parents were crying now as well. "It's us who never wanted to hurt you," said her mother. "We thought we were doing the right thing. We never wanted to bring up your life before because we didn't want to make you relive the horrors, but maybe that was wrong because it also didn't let you relive the happiness either."

We added to the conversation by saying, "And we think Carmen needed to relive the horrors with you there to support her through it. The truth is, she has been reliving them all alone for all these years." Carmen nodded affirmatively and continued to cry.

". . . And this business that we want you to be white. We know you're not white, but who thinks about these things . . . We don't care what color you are, we love you," Mr. Brody said.

"But you are a part of this family, and this is a white family. That's all we meant," Mrs. Brody added.

Mrs. Brody's statement was a complicated one. It conveyed a mixed message. If Carmen truly was a part of the Brody family, as they claimed, and if they accepted that she was a person of color, then they could not be a white family. They were a biracial family. To insist that they were a white family suggested they really did not see Carmen as a member of the family, or it meant that they refused to see her true racial identity. When we made this overt, the Brodys sat stunned. They had never thought of it is this way. For the first time, their deeply held racial beliefs were being unearthed where they would have to examine them up close.

Carmen, feeling somewhat more empowered now, provided them with several examples of things they had said over the years that reinforced the idea that they needed to see her as white. Mrs. Brody began crying hysterically while Mr. Brody tensed up. This was deeply disturbing to both, but they could not avoid the painful truth for long. What ensued was a long, intense conversation about their racial differences and their racial beliefs. In the end, the Brodys could not take back or instantaneously erase the part of them that did need Carmen to be white, but they were able to have the first moments of honesty about their position. This was the beginning of an exploration process that would eventually lead to the types of transformations this family so desperately needed. It also had the powerful effect of liberating Carmen from the shackles of her silence. Simply being able to express herself directly relieved a huge weight from her shoulders. It didn't change some of her parent's prejudices, but it was a relief to have her deepest, most-inner perceptions validated. She no longer had to worry that she was crazy, or hide herself. At long last Carmen and her parents were emerging from the shadows, and this was the beginning of a bridge of true connectedness among all three of them.

Carmen finally was able to tell her parents about her painful experiences in school and why she had never felt the freedom to share these with them. Her parents were deeply troubled to learn all of this and became overwhelmed with feelings of guilt. Part of the therapy involved helping them access enough strength to support Carmen while she shared these secrets, while providing the Brodys with support as well. We offered the family solace by reiterating that the Brodys acted as they did out of love. Maybe they had not made the best choices, but they always did what they believed was best for Carmen.

"What more proof of your love is there than the fact that you have sat here in this session and been so open and honest, even though this has been deeply painful. This is a powerful gift you have given your daughter."

Ultimately, the Brodys just wanted to be good parents. Therefore, it was important for them to hear that they were giving Carmen something valuable through their willingness to listen and to try to be honest with her. If this was a way of being good parents to their daughter, then they could survive the difficulty of this session and would be better for it.

As the primary community in Carmen's life grew stronger, we also needed to help Carmen and her family take steps to establish a strong sense of community at the extended and cultural levels. One of the ways we did this was by engaging Carmen in a series of dialogues about her cultural identity. We encouraged her to write out her story and to express her feelings about her experiences and her identity in a journal. Once she became comfortable with this, we gradually encouraged her to transform some of her writings into an essay for school, which she read aloud in one of her classes. The therapeutic effect this had was tremendous. By telling her story "out loud," she was once again freeing an incarcerated part of herself. Moreover, several students in her class reached out to her as a result of hearing her essay. This was the first time she had friends that she could speak to openly about who she was, and the joys and pains she had experienced. Eventually, Carmen even approached her parents about transferring to another school with more students of color, and she expressed her strong desire to major in Latin American studies in college. These were all critical steps in the restoration of a strong, healthy sense of community at all three levels in Carmen's life.

CONCLUSION

This chapter presented a variety of strategies designed to promote the restoration of community in the lives of adolescents at the primary, extended, and cultural levels. At the primary level disruptions in parent–adolescent relationships tend to be especially damaging. As a result, parents have a responsibility to take specific actions to repair ruptures in their relationships within their teens. Ten suggestions were provided in this chapter to support parents in doing this. Therapists also play a vital role in promoting the restoration of community at the primary level. First, when therapists build a trusting and caring relationship with adolescent clients, this functions as form of primary community. Secondly, there are specific steps that therapists can follow during four successive stages of therapy to facilitate reparations in parent–adolescent relationships. At the extended level parents and therapists can promote the restoration of community by recognizing and intervening when adolescents become involved in negative social groups. Conversely, parents and therapists can assume a proactive role in encouraging teens to develop constructive peer relationships and positive social networks. Teachers play an especially vital role in promoting the restoration of community at this level since school is one of the most salient extended community contexts. Finally, at the cultural level, there are two major ways that adults can promote the restoration of community. The first is by helping adolescents feel pride and confidence about the different dimensions of their (cultural) identity. The second involves assuming an active role in confronting the social forces that contribute to oppression in terms of race, gender, ethnicity, religion, sexual orientation, class, and so forth.

CHAPTER 9

• • • • • • •

Rehumanizing Loss

Darryl's mother had repeatedly chosen to feed her veins with heroin instead of feeding him. Hunger was a constant companion throughout his childhood. Sometimes he went for days at a time enduring the constant ache of an empty stomach. His yearnings for food and the aches of hunger were often unbearable. Trapped in pain, the only way Darryl could survive was by blocking it out. He needed to find a way not to feel what he was feeling. "I used to tell myself I didn't feel hungry. I'd say it over and over again as a way of convincing myself. Eventually I started to believe it. It was like magic."

Darryl used the "magic" he had learned as a child to cope with more than just the hunger in his belly. He also used it to block out the hunger in his heart and soul. The sustenance Darryl was deprived of as a child involved more than just his breakfast or dinner. He also was deprived of emotional sustenance, of the love and affirmation his young heart and soul needed to grow strong and healthy. As a child who was starved of love, Darryl learned how to block out the aching pain created by his emotional hunger. Darryl's way of blocking out the pain of the losses he suffered as a child is a common response. Most people engage in various degrees of repression and denial in response to the overwhelming pain that is generated by experiences with loss. Initially this "blocking out" is a natural part of the healing process. Immediately after a loss has been suffered, it is common to "go numb." A person's entire emotional system shuts down as a form of protection against enormous and potentially debilitating hurt. If however, a person remains emotionally "shut down," disassociated from his or her suffering in perpetuity, problems eventually arise. Without

214

feeling one's pain, healing cannot occur. Hence, those who remain emotionally disconnected from their pain remain wounded and un-healed. This is the case with many of the violent adolescents with whom we work.

Violent adolescents are individuals who have experienced painful losses in their lives—losses that were never healed. Unhealed loss is synonymous with unacknowledged loss. We use the term "acknowl-edged" in a very specific way to refer to an integrated state of cognitive *and* emotional recognition of loss. Those who are able to acknowledge their losses are able to intellectually as well as emotionally recognize and deal with the reality of what they have lost. Unacknowledged loss is the antithesis of acknowledged loss.

When loss remains unacknowledged, it is dehumanized. In other words, loss is stripped of its meaning. The dehumanization of loss is the "loss of all losses"—it is the "mega-loss." When loss is dehuman-ized, the potential for violence increases exponentially. For this rea-son, a critical aspect of addressing adolescent violence must involve the rehumanization of loss, which begins with acknowledgment.

Acknowledgment is an essential step in the rehumanization of loss and the healing process. Unless a person is able to consciously identify what has been lost and emotionally confront and work through the associated feelings, healing cannot occur. Healing re-quires a willingness to confront not only the loss experience but all the attendant emotional baggage as well. To heal, a person must be aware of the wounds that he or she bears and must be able to struggle with all the feelings that inevitably exist in relation to those wounds. There is no healthy way to avoid the agony of loss. Healing can only occur by "walking through the fire." This is why acknowledgment—the capacity to understand what has been lost and to emotionally con-front and work through—is so crucial. For this reason, acknowledg-ment is at the center of the rehumanization (hence, healing) process.

ACKNOWLEDGMENT BEGINS WITH A RELATIONSHIP

Acknowledgment is a relational process. On the one hand, adoles-cents need to be able to acknowledge their losses to themselves. How-ever, experiencing acknowledgment from others is also necessary. In fact, it is the lack of acknowledgment from others that forms the basis of the dehumanization of loss. As Darryl stated: "It didn't seem to me that anyone cared how I felt. Used to be that I would feel bad about things, but no one else seemed to feel bad about any of it. It was like no one else seemed to think anything was wrong. After a while I started to think that maybe there isn't anything wrong—maybe this is just how it is."

What Darryl was describing was the way his losses went unacknowledged by those around him. They acted as if nothing has been lost, as if no tragedy or injustice had occurred. This lack of acknowledgment from others was the beginning of the dehumanization of loss, that is, the process of stripping loss of its meaning. Over time, Darryl began to respond to his losses in the same way that he perceived those around him responding—as if they were unimportant. Hence, the dehumanization of Darryl's losses and his inability to acknowledge them was rooted in his relationships with others and their lack of acknowledgment. For this reason, acknowledging and rehumanizing loss must begin with a secure, trusting relationship between an adolescent and a caring adult. It is through these kinds of relationships that teens receive the critical acknowledgment from others that is a necessary precondition for their acknowledging their losses to themselves.

The importance of a secure, trusting relationship between an adult and an adolescent cannot be overstated. Only when a foundation of basic trust exists will adolescents disclose the details of their lives that reveal the various ways in which they have suffered losses. Moreover, acknowledgment will only be meaningful to the extent that the adolescents have trust in the person offering it. While there is no magical formula that can be relied upon to go establish a secure, trusting relationship with an adolescent, there are several general points that we believe are helpful to keep in mind.

Keepin' It Real

We have heard this phrase so often from the adolescents we work with that we couldn't imagine writing this book without honoring the concept. For adolescents, to *keep it real* means to be your natural self. When one "keeps it real," there is no room for pretense, false platitudes, or fakery. *Keepin' it real* is to proudly and publicly proclaim that "I am what I am . . . What you see is what you get . . . and you can count on me to not play games with you." For many youth, not only is it important for them to *keep it real* with others, but it is also imperative for others to do so with them as well.

For those of us working with violent and aggressive adolescents, *Keepin' it real* is crucial. When our work fails to meet this unspoken and invisible standard for relating, trust is impossible to achieve. Building trust requires us to be as authentic and transparent as possible. Adolescents are experts at detecting fakery. They are neither impressed nor amused by our exaggerated efforts to look or talk cool, or to demonstrate that we really get it. Our relentless efforts to get them to "open up, emote, or participate" often leave them questioning the genuineness of our motives. They invariably become more distant, guarded, and suspicious.

Keepin' it real, within the context of our work, means that we demonstrate the genuine ability to relate to adolescents as "human beings to human beings." It means that we talk to them rather than talk down to them, or at them. It also means that we make a continual and concerted effort to critically examine ourselves so that we know what our strengths, weaknesses, insecurities, etc., are with regard to the work that we do with violent and aggressive adolescents. The degree to which we understand ourselves and can regulate our own anxieties, and risk exposing our own humanity, plays a key role in helping adolescents to risk opening themselves up.

Expect to Be Rebuffed

Working with violent and aggressive adolescents is high-effort, immediate-perpetual-output, delayed-outcome, but rewarding work. It is also work that is often laced with sometimes feisty, sometimes passive, noncompliance—with endless opportunities for rejection. It takes an appreciable amount of time, effort, and patience before most adolescents will open up. In the interim, is it incumbent upon us to remain respectfully persistent in our efforts to reach out and engage our violent and aggressive adolescents. Making numerous thwarted and unreciprocated efforts on behalf of the adolescents we serve is a part of the rough terrain where much of this work takes place. It is important to continue in spite of being continually rebuffed. Respectful persistence is essential. Even when our repeated gestures to establish a connection with a hard-to-reach adolescent go unrewarded, we do not allow this to fracture our hope. When we have respectfully persisted in the face of constant rejection, our efforts have usually been rewarded in the long run. We have learned to trust that if we just keep on talking, keep on reaching out—even as they rebuff us—ultimately, at some point, even the most untrusting and skeptical young person will take a risk and reach back to grab the hand we have extended.

Be Active

One technique we find useful when it comes to talking with adolescents in ways that help them to open up is described at length by William Pollack, author of *Real Boys*. Pollack (1998) writes about the importance of engaging young people (focusing on boys in particular) in activities that they find enjoyable as a means of helping them to relax and eventually open up. Whether it's a round of H-O-R-S-E on the basketball court, drawing pictures, playing a favorite video game, baking cookies, painting one's nails, hiking through the woods, or playing catch, when young boys and girls are busy focusing on an activity they find pleasurable, it puts them at ease. It facilitates a sense of mastery and security that is necessary before one can risk emotional vulnerability. We are strong advocates of engaging adolescents in activities that they enjoy as a foundation for easing them into a casual conversation that will eventually invite a deeper, more vulnerable sharing of inner thoughts, feelings, and experiences.

Read between the Lines

As young people begin to express parts of themselves and their stories to us, it is vital that we have the awareness to detect the losses they have suffered, even when these are not overtly labeled as such. Learning to read between the lines to identify losses, even where they have not been directly stated, is integral to this stage of intervention. We have found that the more we focus on loss in our work with violent and aggressive adolescents, the easier it gets to identify losses that are not overtly stated. Part of this process has been greatly facilitated by our ongoing efforts to remain cognizant of the range of experiences that adolescents have that can be lightning rods for loss. It might be helpful to review Chapter 4 and the section that outlined the 10 different types of loss. This section is critical because it demonstrates numerous ways in which adolescents experience loss—from the most obvious losses (i.e., the death or abandonment of a parent) to the least obvious (i.e., the loss of hope or dignity). Our capacity to assist adolescents with the rehumanization process is greatly facilitated by our ability to think broadly and complexly about loss and the numerous ways in which it can be experienced.

THE COGNITIVE DIMENSION
OF ACKNOWLEDGMENT

The awareness and recognition of losses can vary quite significantly among adolescents. Some possess a cognitive awareness of their losses. Intellectually they recognize and can articulate verbally what they have lost. Emotionally, however, they remain utterly detached from their pain. Consider, for example, Timothy, who was aware of the loss of his father's love; Carmen, who could tell us the first time we met her how she had lost her parents and her connection to her cultural identity; and Daquon, who could describe, with minimal prodding, the death of his father. On a superficial level, each of them was able to cognitively acknowledge their loss very early on in our work together, but none of them was able to do so emotionally. They could not access and connect with the pain, grief, or rage they felt directly in relation to these very concrete losses. Hence, while they could verbally identify some of their losses, they were unable to do so emotionally.

For other adolescents, their lack of acknowledgment is much more pervasive. Not only are they emotionally disconnected from their pain, but they are cognitively, as well. This is the situation with most of the adolescents with whom we work. Early on in our work, we used to ask adolescents directly, "What serious losses have you experienced in your life?" Most would sit blank-faced, staring off into space, wondering what foreign language we were speaking. Eventually they would shrug their shoulders and say, "I don't know . . . None, I guess." Given the magnitude of losses that characterized so many of their lives, responses like these were hard to fathom. But, as unbelievable as they seemed, it was clear that these responses were genuine. Most of these kids simply did not think about their lives in terms of loss. Not only were they emotionally disconnected from the pain of their losses, cognitively they exhibited a virtual lack of recognition of the loss in their lives. In situations such as these, before loss can be acknowledged and rehumanized, it is necessary to help adolescents become aware, cognitively, of what they have lost. An expedition to uncover and identify loss must be undertaken.

The Loss Diagram

The loss diagram is a tool that we developed to identify and track the magnitude of losses experienced by adolescents throughout their lives. The diagram is designed to depict loss, graphically, which helps to promote a cognitive acknowledgment of one's situation or circumstances.

The Exploratory Interview: Uncovering and Identifying Losses

When utilizing the loss diagram, an exploratory interview that is designed to uncover and identify adolescents' losses is a good starting point. Since this is usually very delicate and sensitive work, the mechanics of how the interview is conducted must be attended to carefully. For all practical purposes it should not appear as if the adolescent is being interviewed—but, rather, is participating in a casual conversation. Most adolescents tend to be quite guarded when they are expected to talk about things that hurt them. Except in rare instances, most will not simply provide a list of losses upon request. Therefore, questions that are too direct—that seem like they are part of an interview—are likely to engender a defensive response. This is where creativity and poise are important, because a strictly "head-on" approach is likely to fail. Asking, for example, "Can you please tell me about the losses in your life" will probably not produce the sought-for information.

Another reason why a "head-on" approach is likely to be ineffective is because in many instances adolescents do not even recognize their losses. In such cases, it is impossible to identify an experience that remains hidden from one's own view. Their inability to generate answers about their life experiences can often leave the adolescents feeling stupid and further devalued. Consequently, even when assuming a "just plain talking" approach, our experiences have taught us that it is helpful to take an indirect pathway to uncovering and identifying the losses an adolescent has suffered.

It is impossible to provide a foolproof guide that can be replicated in every situation with every adolescent. At some point, one's own experience and intuition must provide the ultimate direction for talking with adolescents. But in addition to the invaluable guidance that experience and intuition provide, we begin the loss diagram process by utilizing the following Exploratory Interview Guide, which contains questions designed to identify losses in the lives of adolescents.

- "Who were your friends in first grade? Who was your best friend?"
- "What did you and (name of best friend) do for fun back in those

days?" [assessing what was important to the adolescent as clues about what might have been lost]

- "When you were in first grade, where did you live and where did you go to school?"
- "Who helped you get ready for school in the morning?"
- "Back in first grade, how did you get to school?"
- "How did *(name of best friend)* get to school? "
- "Who did you look forward to seeing in school?"
- "Who was home after school was over?"
- "Back when *(name)* was your best friend, what family members do you remember the most?" [shifting from peers to family]
- "What family members were you closest to when you were in first grade?"
- "What was it like at home when you were in the first grade? How did everyone get along with each other? What were your relationships like with those family members?"
- "Do you still live in the same place you lived in when you were in the first grade?"
- "Do you still live in the same neighborhood as when you were in the first grade?" [shifting from family to community]
- "How often do you still pass by the school you went to in first grade?"
- "Who was your best friend when you were 10 years old?" [If this person is different from best friend in first grade, inquire about what happened to that person.]
- "Who else were your friends when you were 10 and in the fifth grade?"
- "Okay, so now you're __ years old? [shifting from the past to the present, starting with friends]
- "How many friends from first grade do you still have today?"
- "Are you still friends with *(name of best friend at age 10)*?"
- "Of the friends that you lost contact with from fifth grade, what happened?"
- "How many friends have you lost due to drugs? moving away? some other reason?"
- "How many friends did you have that died? How did they die?"
- "Tell me about your relationships with each of your family members now." [shifting from friends to family]
- "How many family members have you lost due to drugs? divorce or separation? moving away? because they just don't get along with you?"

- "How many family members do you know who died in your lifetime? How did they die?"
- "As you reflect on this conversation and the diagram we have constructed [see next section for examples], what does it say to you about your experiences with loss? What thoughts and feelings have been brought up?"
- "Which of these losses have you had a chance to mourn? How did you do that and what effect did this have? And which losses have remained unacknowledged or unmourned, and what effect has this had in your life?"

One of the first points to bear in mind is that when we talk about uncovering and identifying losses, we think about this as a "fact-finding mission." Because this occurs early on in our relationship with an adolescent, we are careful not to push too quickly at trying to unearth feelings associated with losses. Especially with boys, it is generally not a good idea to name emotions or make them too obvious too quickly, because this tends to be very threatening, especially with traumatized teens. Also, when working cross-racially, moving slowly is very strongly indicated. Instead of opening them up further, moving too quickly toward emotions often shuts them down. So, initially we start slowly and focus primarily on uncovering the "facts" associated with their loss stories. Our goal is to reconstruct the events, dates, and details that make up their unique loss stories.

The process of gathering facts and reconstructing loss stories is facilitated by the questions contained in the Exploratory Interview Guide. Notice that the questions begin with friends as opposed to family, because often it's safer for adolescents to talk about their peer relationships first. We also begin with an earlier period in time—for example, when the adolescent was 5 or 6, just about the time when he or she was starting school for the first time and around the time when most people have their first clear childhood memories. As specified in the Exploratory Interview Guide, the nature of our initial questions are rather bland and circumspect, as in one of the early questions, such as "Who was your best friend when you were in first grade?" In most cases, a question like this elicits little panic. It tends to be low-risk, which is important for establishing trust and a sense of safety early on in the conversation. Of course, if a question like this appears to arouse a great deal of emotion, this also becomes critical information (we will say more about this in the section titled "How To Deal with Strong Emotional Reactions").

A question about a best friend at age 6 is important for beginning to construct a picture of the adolescent's early relationship network. This is the beginning stage of finding out who was important to this person early on in his or her life. For this reason, we pay specific attention to finding out people's names (i.e., "What was the name of your best friend when you were 6?"). Questions like "How did you get to and from school?," "Who helped you get ready for school in the morning?," and "Who was home when you got home from school?" are further ways of gathering information about an adolescent's early relationship network and what his or her life was like on a daily basis. Certainly these don't get at the whole story, but the answers to each of these questions contain vital clues that the interviewer/listener must pay close attention to at all times.

Gradually the questions shift to a later point in life, around age 10. To maintain the continuity of the conversation, the next set of questions makes explicit ties with the information that has been gathered up until that point. Hence, asking "When you were 10, was _____ still your best friend?" is a way of finding out what happened in this person's life over the course of the 4 or 5 years between age 6 and 10. If he or she remained best friends with the same person, it implies continuity, which is important information to know. It points to the saliency of that relationship. On the other hand, if one's best friend changed between age 6 and 10, it would be important to find out how that happened and why. Certainly it is not uncommon for children to change best friends on a frequent basis. But the end of one "best friendship" may be linked to loss issues (i.e., perhaps one's family moved to another area, or maybe there was a conflict and subsequent distancing between friends). This is the type of information the interviewer/listener must gradually uncover. Everything is information, and no information is a disposable. Every small detail, no matter how seemingly irrelevant, is a clue about someone's life. We treat all information as valuable. Nothing is irrelevant, from our perspective.

As the questions continue, they begin to shift by gradually moving forward through time, working up to the present moment. They also vacillate in and out between the adolescent's nonfamily and family relations. For example, the question that focuses on school ("Who did you look forward to seeing at school?") is followed by questions that hint at one's family/home life ("Who got you ready for school in the morning?," "How did you get to and from school?," and "Who was home when you got home from school?"). Each of these questions, on the surface, seems to be about school, but collectively they also are ways of gathering information about the adolescent's home life when he or she was young.

As the facts of an adolescent's life are gathered, and as the pieces of his or her loss story start to unfold, it is important to direct the conversation in a way that helps the adolescent to start to think about these "facts" in terms of loss. This may seem like an obvious point, but its importance cannot be overstated. The reality is that most teens do not think about their lives in terms of loss. This simply is not a framework that they use to make sense of their worlds. This is why most teens cannot answer a direct question about what they have lost. This is where a lot of supportive assistance is needed. During the process of gathering the facts of an adolescent's life, it is important to ask strategic questions that serve the purpose of directing them to think about the facts in terms of loss. For example, we routinely ask:

- "How did your life change after *(whatever the event was)* happened?"
- "How did the value or meaningfulness of *(whatever person, event, or thing that was important to the adolescent)* change after *(the change-producing event or experience)* occurred?"

These questions are designed to direct an adolescent's attention to the concept of loss. By asking adolescents to contemplate how something changed in response to a disruptive event or experience, it invites them they to think in terms of loss.

Organizing and Visually Depicting Loss

Whether one uses the Exploratory Interview Guide or some other method for uncovering and identifying loss, the information that has been gathered about the adolescent's story of loss must be organized in a comprehensive way. Wherever possible, we construct a loss diagram as a way of organizing adolescents' stories of loss visually. We have found that there is something remarkably potent about "seeing" the picture of one's loss.

The construction of a loss diagram begins by mapping out an adolescent's relationship system. A strong bias that we hold is that individuals experience their world relationally. Our sense of who we are as people is defined in relationship to others—how we perceive others and how we believe others perceive us. Because we believe human life is essentially a relational experience, we believe the concept of loss is fundamentally tied to our relationships with others and the world around us. When one suffers the loss of a family member or friend, the relational nature of the loss is obvious. However, while more difficult to detect at first, intangible losses also are relationally defined. Consider the loss of respect, which is an intangible loss. Respect is a relational concept. People strive to earn the respect of others. Even when one loses respect for one's self, inevitably the events related to this loss of self-respect involve other people. Perhaps one allowed him- or herself to be treated poorly by a friend. In a situation like this, the person feels a loss of respect for him- or herself that ultimately is tied to feeling disrespected by the friend. Hence, issues of respect are relational. This is the case with all forms of loss. Because we as humans are relational beings, it is impossible to identify a single experience that does not reveal the relational dimensions of our existence.

The loss diagram is designed to recognize the relational dimension of life and loss. Because we believe all loss is tied to relationships, we depict losses in an individual's life in terms of their relationship systems. By using circles (to denote females), squares (to denote males), and lines (to denote relationships), a loss diagram constructs an individual's relational world. After the basic relationships that characterize an individual's life are mapped out, the next step in constructing a loss diagram involves mapping out where the various losses have occurred. This is accomplished by using a combination of colors and brief verbal descriptors to identify where various losses have occurred throughout a person's life/relationship system (see Figure 9.1).

We arbitrarily use the color blue to denote physical/tangible loss and red to denote emotional/intangible loss. Certainly, it is true that all physical losses involve some degree of emotional loss as well. Our distinction between physical and emotional losses is designed to capture the complexity of loss with the understanding that some part of the distinction we make is artificial. We direct the reader's attention to Figures 9.1, 9.2, and 9.3, which reflect the loss diagrams of Timothy Ryan, Carmen Brody, and Daquon Jackson, respectively.

THE EMOTIONAL DIMENSION OF ACKNOWLEDGMENT

Once adolescents become aware of their losses cognitively, the second dimension of acknowledgment involves connecting emotionally to the feelings associated with loss.

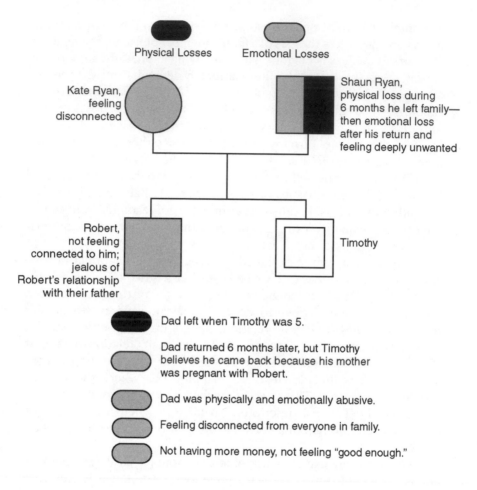

FIGURE 9.1. Timothy Ryan's loss diagram.

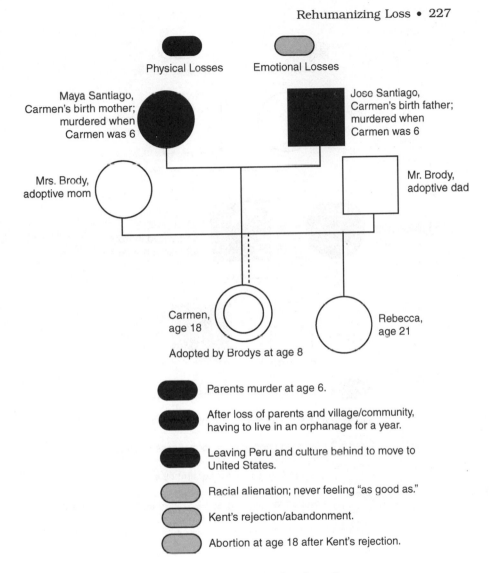

FIGURE 9.2. Carmen Brody's loss diagram.

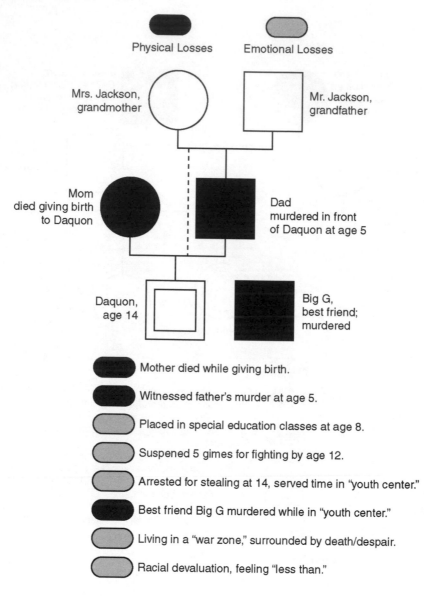

FIGURE 9.3. Daquon Jackson's loss diagram.

Connecting Loss to Rage/Violence

Rage is one of the first emotions adolescents access as they begin to connect with their losses emotionally. As our model indicates, rage plays a pivotal role in the violence that many adolescents exhibit. Rage, more than any other emotion, bridges violence and loss. Rage is both a response to the pain and injustice of loss and a catalyst for violence. Yet, when loss is unacknowledged, the relationship between loss, rage, and violence remains invisible. As a result, adolescents who suffer from unacknowledged loss experience a type of "free-floating rage," that is, they feel a generalized sense of rage that they are unable to connect with any specific origin. Gradually, however, as loss becomes acknowledged, the roots of their rage become increasingly clear. For this reason, as adolescents begin to recognize their losses cognitively, one of the first emotions they connect with is rage. The generalized rage they felt but never understood now becomes focused around their emerging awareness of the losses they have suffered. As adolescents begin to cognitively recognize their losses, they start to understand the basis for their rage. As they begin to relate to the basis of their rage, they begin to recognize the emotional dimension of loss. Hence, rage plays a pivotal role in illuminating the relationship between loss and violence and in helping adolescents to begin to acknowledge loss emotionally.

Often it doesn't require anything sophisticated to draw out and build upon the natural connections that exist between loss, rage, and violence, and to use rage as a starting point for helping teens to acknowledge loss on an emotional level. One of the first things we routinely say to adolescents is simply, "I'm seeing here all the things you've lost, and I'm realizing how unfair this was. It certainly helps me to understand why you've been so enraged." A basic, straightforward comment like this can go a long way toward highlighting the relationship between loss, rage, and violence, and toward normalizing feelings of rage. This is the beginning of redefining adolescents from "bad" to "hurt" (as in the case of those who externalize their violence) or from "sick" to "hurt" (which is the key with adolescents who internalize their violence). Making explicit the ties between experiences with loss, rage, and violence is a step in the direction of humanizing these adolescents so that their troubling behaviors can begin to make sense within the context of their life experiences and stories of loss. These connections create a critical opening for the acknowledgment of other emotions associated with loss. For more on working with the relationships between loss, rage, and violence, see Chapter 10.

Encouraging Other Emotions Associated with Loss

Having opportunities to express rage and having this emotion normalized can greatly facilitate the eventual release of other strong emotions associated with loss. Once adolescents are able to "release" their rage and to have it validated, it clears the air, making it easier for them to gain access to emotions like grief, shame, and fear. Of course, this is not an absolute. Some struggle tremendously when it comes to connecting with emotions. Even after a large release of rage, they still closely guard against the expression of more vulnerable emotions. Having been traumatized by a plethora of unacknowledged losses, many adolescents have learned, even without fully understanding why, how to exchange raw vulnerability for feigned invincibility. In fact, some are so emotionally blocked that even expressions of rage are difficult to express. They retain all of their emotions. In situations like these, it is imperative not to be seduced by the "cool pose," stone-faced physical presentations. It is important to recognize these "appearances" for what they are—evidence of feigned invincibility that hides an often frightened and wounded child. The nuances of this aspect of loss work require determination, creativity, and patience, all of which are necessary to create a context in which adolescents can express their emotions freely.

Using Symbolism, Metaphors, and Stories

It can be extremely difficult to get adolescents to connect with emotions, especially vulnerable ones. For this reason, we have found it useful to use symbolism, metaphors, and stories as pathways toward helping them focus on their losses and connect with the associated pain. For example, movies can be a powerful medium for connecting teens with the pain of their losses. We have successfully used movies such as *Boyz 'n the Hood, Mi Familia, The Outsiders, Higher Learning, Girl, Interrupted, What's Eating Gilbert Grape?, American Beauty,* and *Boys Don't Cry* as catalysts to help adolescents reconnect with their emotions. The following is a sample of the types of questions that we typically ask in our adolescent group settings:

- "What was the basic story about?"
- "What messages about life did this movie teach?"
- "Which character did you identify with the most, and why?"
- "Which character did you identify with the least, and why?"
- "What scene in the movie affected you most powerfully, and why?"

We try to tailor the movies we select to the individual adolescents with whom we work, based on our knowledge of their personal stories and unique identities. We draw from our experiences with them as a way of making educated guesses about what specific movie might be most effective at tapping into a given adolescent's loss issues. Most of the time, our efforts have been successful. However, there have also been moments where we missed the mark and did not gain what we had hoped to from the experience. Our motto is "Nothing ventured, nothing gained." There are even instances when we have stumbled upon movies that have unexpectedly connected with an adolescent's loss experiences. One such instance occurred recently when one of us (TAL) was watching three children for the day as a favor to their parents. Two of the children, a brother and sister, were ages 7 and 8; the third child, who was 13, was their cousin. After we had painted, played kickball, had ice cream, and given the dog a bath, I was exhausted and needed some "down-time." They excitedly elected to watch the movie *The Lion King*, one of the few I had on hand. When the movie was over, I decided to engage them in a discussion that followed the questions outlined above. The conversation was flowing freely, and I was impressed with the excellent and enthusiastic responses I was getting from each of them. I was surprised, however, when I asked which scene in the movie most affected them, and I turned first to Tia, the 13-year-old, and observed her obvious emotion. I had just assumed that she was watching as a way of going along with the other kids; as I generally found her to be compliant most of the time. I didn't really expect that *The Lion King* would be all that interesting to a 13-year-old, but clearly the movie had captured something inside of her.

Tia appeared extremely sullen and introspective, and when she answered my question she began to cry. I moved closer to her and just sat with her as she tearfully explained that "The scene that got to me the most was when Simba's father died. That was so sad." Because I knew Tia's history, I realized instantly what was happening for her. Three years earlier she had lost her father. He died when his car was hit by a drunk driver. Tia was identifying with Simba who, as a young lion cub, also tragically lost his father in an unexpected accident. Since Simba's story was the vehicle for connecting Tia to her emotions, I continued to use it. Although I knew she was feeling the pain of losing her father, I stayed with Simba's story. I said to her: "Yes, that was a terrible thing that happened to Simba's father. What do you think Simba was feeling when that happened?" Tia sobbed as she explained: "He felt like his heart was broken. He never felt anything as sad . . . ever! He felt all alone. He missed his dad more than anything, more than anything. He just wanted his dad to come back."

Simba's story became a powerful vehicle for Tia to tell her loss story. She was describing her own experience, but through Simba—a connection I eventually made explicit by saying, "You seem to really understand how Simba feels." She nodded in agreement. "As someone who has gone through something similar, I guess you can really understand how terrible he must have felt." She nodded again and eventually began to talk more directly about the sadness she still felt intensely, 3 years after her father's death. Once the loss issues and the associated emotions have been triggered, it is critical to offer emotional support, validation, and empathy. In the case of Tia, after she began to cry and ultimately talk about her father, I spent the next hour talking with her about her feelings of loss and grief. It turned out to be an extremely powerful experience that was facilitated by an unexpected catalyst, *The Lion King*.

Movies are only one way of using symbolism, metaphors, and stories to help adolescents connect with their loss experiences. Another common medium we utilize are songs. We have yet to meet an adolescent who doesn't love some type of music, whether it's rap, country, gospel, rock, blues, reggae, or even classical. Whatever an adolescent's musical tastes might be, we have found that music facilitates an instant pathway to an individual's emotional nerve center. For this reason, we often invite adolescents to share with us their favorite songs or musical pieces, and we ask them to explain to us why this song or that piece of music is meaningful to them. Some of the most passionate, introspective, and vulnerable disclosures from adolescents occurred in response to the question "What song would you pick to say something about your life, and why?"

Darryl didn't hesitate for a moment:

"I would pick my favorite Tupac song, 'Me Against the World.' That song says it all for me. Since I was little that's the way it's been. Ain't nobody been there to take care of me. I had to make do for myself. Even when my moms was around, it was like I was still alone. And all those years I lived on the streets, I had to always watch my own back because I couldn't count on no one else to back me up. I've had to be my mother, father, and best friend all at once, but I did it. Like the brother is saying, it ain't easy. It's tough, but you do what you have to, and I did."

Embedded in Darryl's explanation of why he chose 'Me Against the World' as the song that says the most about him is his story of loss. Using the song as his vehicle, he tells the story of a young boy who grew up parentless, who felt friendless and unloved, and yet who—in spite of his alienation and isolation, his loneliness and despair—learned to fend for himself and survive. The song provided a powerful opportunity for Darryl to "give voice" to his story of loss, suffering, and survival.

The use of symbolism, metaphors, and stories can be powerful aids in helping teens identify and emotionally connect with the pain of their losses. Once this occurs, it is critical that we, as adults—in whatever capacity we are interacting with teens—find ways to remain emotionally present with them, to mirror back that we recognize what they have lost, and to convey compassion and empathy for their pain.

REHUMANIZING LOSS WITH VALIDATION AND EMPATHY

Validation and empathy are essential to the process of rehumanizing loss. Once losses and the feelings associated with them are identified, validation and empathy should be used liberally and consistently. When used genuinely, both validation and empathy play an instrumental role in reestablishing trust and fostering a delicately formed emotional bond.

The process of rehumanizing loss requires not only validation and empathy but also the ability to convey compassion toward adolescents. Extending empathy, compassion, and validation to adolescents allows then to experience dimensions of a relationship that may be alien to them, especially on a consistent basis. As stated previously, the difficulty many adolescents have acknowledging their losses is rooted in a lack of acknowledgment that they receive from those around them. Remember how Darryl explained that everyone around him acted as if nothing much had happened. In spite of the trauma he had endured, the world around him carried on with "business as usual." Darryl's inability to acknowledge his losses to himself began with the lack of acknowledgment he perceived from those around him. Before adolescents can feel compassion for themselves, they need to experience someone else feeling it for them as a way of giving them permission, as a way of modeling what it looks like.

To adequately convey empathy and compassion toward another person, one must genuinely possess these feelings. They cannot be faked. Yet, even when these feelings are genuinely present, they must also be explicitly expressed. It is a huge mistake to assume others intuitively know what we think and feel and to therefore minimize the significance of expressing thoughts and feelings directly. We can't begin to count the number of times we have sat in therapy with families and heard a parent say, "But don't you know that I love you? . . . that I'm proud of you? . . . that I'm afraid for you?" And then we look over at their children, who consistently say: "No. You've never said that before. I didn't know you felt that way." Both parties seem mystified. For parents, their feelings seem so obvious to themselves that they just assume their children know how they feel. It doesn't occur to them that they never take the time to actually say how they feel. For adolescents whose parents never tell them how they feel, they are left to infer their parent's feelings based upon their actions. Thus, in the absence of direct verbal expressions of love and caring, every missed basketball game, every night Mom or Dad worked late and was not home for dinner, whenever a parent didn't have time to talk or snapped out, in irritation—all these experiences became signs of not caring.

Even in families where parents do not directly express their feelings but their children somehow intuitively understand and receive them, there is no substitute for the power of hearing it directly. A few weeks ago we worked with an adult woman and her aged father. This woman knew that her father loved her in spite of the fact that he had never told her. And yet, while she knew it, and while she had never doubted his love, when he finally told her, when she finally heard these words at the age of 45, she cried hysterically. Simply "knowing it" cannot match the power of hearing it directly. So, our point is simple: make it explicit! Adults must convey their compassion and empathy toward adolescents directly. Adolescents need to hear an adult say to them in no uncertain terms, "I not only recognize that this happened to you, that you lost _____, which was important to you, but I also realize how incredibly painful this was for you, and that matters to me because I care about you." Teens need to hear from us directly that we recognize their loss and that we care about it . . . that it matters to us.

OPPORTUNITIES FOR MOURNING AND HEALING

An integral part of the rehumanization of loss involves the mourning process. Mourning is fundamentally related to acknowledgment in the sense that one cannot mourn without simultaneously acknowledging loss on an emotional level. Mourning entails working through the emotional stages of loss until one is able to achieve some closure or resolution with respect to the loss.

Elizabeth Kübler-Ross (1970) has identified a five-stage grieving cycle. According to her model, after loss occurs, individuals progressively experience: (1) denial; (2) anger; (3) bargaining; (4) sadness; and finally (5) acceptance. After using this model very effectively with other clients, we attempted to use it in our work with violent and aggressive adolescents. Unfortunately, we quickly discovered that most violent and aggressive youth engage in an abbreviated grieving cycle that results in a type of pseudomourning and pseudoresolution. After a loss has occurred, rather than experiencing the extended grieving cycle that Kübler-Ross identified, many adolescents advance through a much more expedited "cycle" that includes (1) rage, (2) revenge, and (3) (pseudo)resolution. Time and again we have seen adolescents whose immediate response to loss and pain has been overwhelming rage and an almost obsessive need to exact revenge for the injustice they perceive. Unfortunately, the cycle of rage, revenge, and resolution is in part what perpetuates the cycle of youth violence. Every act of violence demands vindication, which is an act of violence that begets vindication and ultimately more violence. So continues the vicious deadly cycle of adolescent violence.

Adolescents are not alone in this orientation toward revenge. They learn it from us, as a society. Capital punishment is an obvious example of the support our society provides for revenge-based approaches to loss and pain. We understand that it is probably normal to desire some form of revenge in the face of a significant loss. However, ultimately the pathway to revenge seldom leads to healing. Executing murderers doesn't bring back their victims. It may feel good in the short run, but in the end the friends and family of the victim are still left with a hole in their lives. They are still left with the unbearable pain that emanates from their loss. At some point, if they are to heal, they will have to confront the messy, excruciating, and complicated ordeal that healing inevitably involves.

The same is true for the adolescents who move all too quickly to respond to the pain of their losses with the rage–revenge–(pseudo)resolution cycle. The "payback" may feel good in the short run, but in the long run it does little to heal their wounds. In our work with adolescents who are violent, we try to be ever mindful of the reality that their violence is a way of coping with the agony of their losses. What these adolescents need most is help in learning how to connect with their feelings so they can embark upon a healing process. This healing process requires many things. It requires the identification of losses, making connections between loss, rage, and violence, encouraging expressions of grief as well as rage, conveying compassion and empathy, and, finally, helping adolescents to engage in a process of mourning. The use of mourning rituals is a way of acknowledging what has been lost, providing a formal opportunity for expressing vulnerable emotions, and a means for "saying good-bye" to what has been lost that can never be regained (Imber Black & Roberts, 1993). Mourning rituals are a way of achieving closure so that the wound can begin to heal and the individual can start to move forward.

We define mourning rituals as a formalized set of behaviors that are executed in a ceremonious manner for the express purpose of acknowledging a specific loss, and honoring the suffering that was experienced in relationship to that loss. Rituals are, by design, exercises in formality and ways of recognizing pain and suffering. A critical component of mourning rituals is that they are most effective when they occur within a community of care and/or when the rituals are a way of solidifying or restoring a community that has been disrupted. While some mourning rituals may involve humor and joy, they must always involve respectfulness, dignity, and paying homage to loss. Above all, mourning rituals are a way of saying "good-bye."

Burial Ceremonies

When adolescents lose someone they loved (whether due to death, abandonment, or some other reason), we often assist them in holding a burial ceremony. One such case involved a 17-year-old girl, Celia, whose father had died when she was only an infant—hence, she never knew him. Raised as an only child by her mother, who never remarried, Celia had lived her whole life yearning for the father she had lost. Part of her healing required finding a way to mourn her loss, a way to honor the image she held in her heart of her father, as well as saying good-bye. To do this we organized a formal ceremony with her and her mother.

During the ceremony Celia read several very powerful entries from her diary, where she had described at length her vision of her father—she described him as he existed in her mind's eye. Doing so was a way of invoking the spirit of her father, and once he had been "summoned forth," we had her speak to the spirit of her father directly. We had her tell him all the things she wanted him to know about what her life had been like without him, how she missed him, and the young woman that she was becoming. She also told to him about the fears and hopes she had for her future and the things that she wished he could be there for to offer support or to share in her joy. She told him how she wanted him to be there to meet her date before her senior prom, to help move into her college dorm for the first time, to hug her when she was sad, to give her fatherly advice when she was confused, to sit with her mother when she graduated from college, and to walk her down the aisle at her wedding. These were all the things she wanted but would never have with him. Finally, she ended by saying good-bye to him. She told him, "I have missed not having you here for all the big and little moments, and I will continue to miss you in the future. But in a way you have always been with me in my heart, so now I can officially say good-bye to you, because I understand that even when you can't be here in the flesh, I know you will always be here in spirit, right by my side." She concluded the ceremony by burying a small box in which she had placed a picture of her father and his watch. She explained that she had held on to this watch as if she was somehow holding on to him. She had been afraid of ever letting it go. But finally, she realized that her father had been with her not through the watch, but in spirit. In this sense, he would always be by her side. But she had to let go of the idea of her father in a physical sense. He was gone and she would never know him. She had to accept this. Burying the photo and the watch was her way of letting go so that she could finally accept her loss, heal, and move forward.

A vital component of the burial ceremony involved the presence of Celia's mother, Rose. Her mother's presence was necessary for several reasons. First, it was a way of strengthening the primary community in Celia's life. Second, her mother's presence was a form of acknowledgement of Celia's loss. Almost all societies have public mourning rituals when someone dies, and in part the public nature of the event is based on the awareness that healing requires some external validation and recognition that one has suffered a loss. In Celia's case, she needed her mother to bear witness to her loss and her mourning process as a critical aspect of acknowledgment. Third, one of the things that had impaired Celia's capacity to mourn her father was the fact that her mother had never truly mourned him and let go. For the past 16 years she too had been holding on in a way that had sabotaged her own mourning process, which therefore affected Celia's. Hence, including Rose in the burial ceremony allowed both mother and daughter to say good-bye and explicitly work on having closure together. Along these lines, Rose also spoke to her deceased husband, sharing with him what it had been like to lose him, to have to raise their daughter without him, how she missed him, how proud she was of Celia, and how she wished he could see the woman she was becoming. She too formally said good-bye and included in the box her wedding band. Both mother and daughter cried hysterically during the burial, but afterward there was a sense of serenity that washed over them. They marked "the gravesite" and agreed that every year they would return together to acknowledge the significance of this date.

Tributes

Another form of mourning ritual involves having adolescents prepare a tribute to someone or something that they have lost. For example, adolescents often write poems or songs memorializing their loss, and they recite or sing these during a formal tribute that is designed to commemorate their loss and to facilitate the process of saying good-bye. We have had adolescents who have made videotapes, written eulogies, painted pictures, and taken photographs that they used to create a commemorative photo essay. We always have them present their work during a formal tribute, and whenever possible we invite others to witness and support the adolescent during the mourning ritual. The idea of a tribute was actually adapted from a type of mourning ritual that many gangs use with their members. Over the years, we have had gang-affiliated adolescents describe very brief quasi-mourning rituals that are prominent within their culture. Unfortunately, many of these often involve drugs and alcohol that from our perspective impede the broader goal of the ritual to promote emotional healing.

Provocative Aids

When we are working with violent and aggressive adolescents in a group setting, we frequently introduce a mourning process by creating a ritual of our own. Typically we do this by either showing a videotape of playing a song that we know has an emotional potency that will inevitably induce deep emotions and facilitate a mourning process within the group. For example, we have a videotape that features a funeral scene with a rap song playing in the background. The song was written by a young man who was expressing deep grief over the death of his little sister, who was gunned down in a drive-by shooting. The song has a haunting rhythm, and the words are filled with intense sadness that beautifully captures the horror and senselessness of her death and the pain this loss has created. In combination with the song, the accompanying visual imagery is haunting—young men carrying a small casket as family and friends stand by, overwhelmed with grief. The scene plays in slow motion, and in black and white, as if to capture the sense that the pain is endless and the loss all-consuming.

When we are working with adolescents in a group who have experienced the death of a peer to a senseless act of violence, this video often has a riveting impact. They relate to it instantly, and it triggers intense emotions that are a vital part of the mourning and healing process. After showing the video, we engage the adolescents in a dialogue. We ask them to share what they are feeling, encourage them to recognize that they have endured individual as well as collective loss, and emphasize the need for them to support one another during this difficult time.

CONCLUSION

The rehumanization of loss is a vital aspect of working with adolescents who are violent. This rehumanization process must begin with acknowledging that losses have been suffered, which begins through relationship. Adolescents will start to open up and explore their losses only if they are able to do so within a safe and trusting relationship. Once such a relationship exists, the first step to rehumanizing loss begins with a cognitive acknowledgement of loss.

One of key strategies we recommend is utilizing a loss diagram. This graphic aid helps to identify and uncover losses, as well as organize and visually depict them. With cognitive acknowledgement, it is possible to then move into emotionally acknowledging loss. Part of this entails connecting loss to rage or violence, encouraging other emotions associated with loss, and using symbolism, metaphors, and stories to assist adolescents in connecting with their feelings. Throughout all of this, it is vital for adults to rehumanize loss with heavy doses of validation and empathy. Ultimately, it is important to assist teens in mourning their losses. One way to do this is through the use of mourning rituals that simultaneously acknowledge what has been lost, allow teens to work through the emotional stages of loss, receive validation from a community of caring others, and ultimately achieve closure by saying "good-bye" to their loss.

CHAPTER 10

· · · · · · · ·

Rechanneling Rage

As discussed at length in Chapter 5, rage is a normal, healthy response to pain and injustice. Difficulties arise when rage is suppressed and denied expression. As a result, it builds in intensity, growing ever more potent and volatile until finally it erupts, often in violent ways. Consequently, our position on rage is that this powerful emotion must have an outlet—it must be expressed. It is not helpful to bury feelings of rage in the naive hope that, if only rage is ignored, it will eventually go away. Since rage is a normal response to pain and injustice that is exacerbated when denied or buried, the issue becomes one of finding constructive ways to channel rage. This is the critical task. Rather than focusing on preventing expressions of rage, our energies are best expended when devoted to inviting expressions of rage and finding healthy, positive ways for it to be channeled.

IDENTIFYING AND INVITING RAGE

How to identify and invite expressions of rage varies with the uniqueness of each individual situation. There are, however, several general tips that we can offer, based upon our work. The first of these involves the importance of *tracking* what adolescents say. It's important to listen closely to what they tell us. If we pay close enough attention, we often discover that they have indirect ways of talking about their rage. If we track the indirect and covert expressions properly, it usually directs us to unexpressed rage. In addition to picking up on and following the clues adolescents give us about their rage, we also recommend responding to them with a combination of *validating* and *zooming in*. It is extremely useful to send messages back to adolescents letting them know that what they're saying is both heard and understood. At the same time, gradually encouraging and directing them toward talking about their rage with greater and greater specificity is also necessary. The following excerpt from a dialogue we had with Darryl illustrates the concepts of tracking, validating, and zooming in.

> THERAPIST: So, when Mr. Weiner sent you to the principal's office, you were so mad you wanted to kill him?
>
> DARRYL: That's right.
>
> THERAPIST: I've noticed that this is something you feel a lot—pissed off. Have you noticed how often you feel pissed?
>
> DARRYL: I never much thought about it before. But, yeah, I guess I do feel pissed a lot, for good reason.
>
> THERAPIST: Yeah, I agree. You've had some tough breaks. A lot of messed-up stuff has happened to you. Could you tell me more about being pissed off?
>
> DARRYL: I don't know what else to say. *(There was a pause, during which time we all just sat there in silence.)* I'm just sick and tired of people thinking they can treat me like shit. I'm not going to just take it. If someone disses me, I'm going to push right back.
>
> THERAPIST: You said you're sick of people treating you like shit. So, who treats you that way? Who pisses you off the most? Who are some of the worst people that you would really like to get back at?

As this excerpt from our dialogue with Darryl indicates, we were able to identify rage by closely following his lead, and we invited him to talk about his rage by reflecting back what we heard and by validating his right to feel pissed off. We also encouraged him to be more specific about feeling "pissed off." For example, we verbally acknowledged his disclosure that he felt so mad he wanted to kill. We punctuated this idea and held it up for further examination by asking him if he noticed how often he feels pissed off. In this way, we not only tracked the idea of his anger but also invited him to be more specific (i.e., "How often do you feel pissed off?"). Darryl continued by saying he had good reason to feel pissed off, which we immediately validated. We followed validation by inviting him to say more about being pissed off. At first he stumbled, saying he didn't know what else to say. We remained silent, trusting that if we didn't jump in too quickly he would come up with more to say, which he did. He mentioned that he was sick of people treating him badly, and he wasn't going to take it anymore. Again, we simply followed what he was saying by inviting him to be more specific (i.e., "Who have you felt most dissed by? Who are you most pissed off at?").

Identifying and inviting the expression of rage is fairly easy with someone like Darryl, who was actively in touch with being "pissed off." This is much harder to do with someone like Rudy, a 14-year-old male client whose rage was very much buried and whose resulting violence was all directed inwardly against himself. Darryl's behavior pointed toward rage in an obvious way (i.e., he had numerous fistfights with other boys, he often shouted and yelled at other kids and adults when he became frustrated, he was prone to using profanity, and he often used expressions like "He pissed me off so much I wanted to kill him" or "She needed a good slap to teach her not to piss me off that way"). But Rudy's rage was not obvious. Rudy was very quiet and withdrawn. He never raised his voice, never used aggressive language, and he never engaged in threatened or actual violence toward others. But Rudy's attempted suicide was a definite act of violence against himself, and it was fueled by all the ingredients identified in our model: devaluation, disruption of community, loss, and, of course, rage. Indeed, Rudy felt a great deal of rage, but it was buried rage, and when the intensity of this contained emotion finally erupted, it imploded inwardly, leading Rudy to lash out violently against himself.

Before adolescents like Rudy can accept an invitation to express their rage, they first need to recognize their own rage. They also need a way of thinking about their experiences that grants them a sense of entitlement to their rage. This is very difficult for adolescents who are prone toward internalization of their rage and subsequent violence. Rage is a righteous emotion. It assumes that an injustice has been suffered. To feel rage, a person has to see him- or herself as an injured party, as someone who has suffered an incontestable and significant wrong. Adolescents like Rudy have difficulty seeing themselves in this way. They believe that there is something about them that is bad and/or wrong and so whatever pain and suffering they have endured, they believe they deserve.

Before we can get adolescents like this to express rage, we first need to help them think about the suffering they have been subjected to as unjust. In Rudy's case, he had known since he was 6 that he was gay, but he never felt the freedom to express this because of strong messages he received from his father and other friends and family members who made generalized anti-gay remarks. Rudy believed that he was sick and that there was something wrong with how he felt. He tried to hide who he was as a way of protecting himself from the scorn and rejection he knew he would receive if others knew he was gay. But Rudy knew. No matter how hard he tried to deny himself, he knew he was gay.

Although he was filled with shame and fear, as a young adolescent whose sexuality was beginning to burgeon, he was compelled to seek out intimate relationships with others. There was another boy in school, Jay, whom Rudy reports that he had a crush on for months. According to Rudy, he was sure Jay felt the same way. One day Jay struck up a conversation with Rudy, and before he knew it the two were becoming intimately involved. One day when Jay was at Rudy's house after school and the two were in his room studying, Jay unexpectedly kissed Rudy. It was a wonderful moment for Rudy—his first kiss—and he was so in love with Jay. It felt incredible. Perhaps because he was so swept away in the magic of the moment, he never heard his father's footsteps outside his door. He never heard his father open the door to his room and walk in on the two boys, forever shattering what had been one of the best moments in Rudy's life.

Rudy stated that he had never seen his father this angry before in his life. "He was fuming. His face turned fire red, and he screamed 'Get your hands off my son, you fucking faggot!'"

All Rudy could remember is that his father lunged at Jay, throwing him against the wall and then picking him up only to push him violently out the door. "Get the hell out of my house, and don't let me ever see your face again!"

Recounting the story to us forced Rudy to relive the experience. He began to shake almost uncontrollably as he fought back tears. "I was horrified! I never moved. I was frozen with fear. My father didn't say a word to me—he left the room, slamming the door behind him. I remained in my room the rest of the day," Rudy painfully recalled. Later that night his father came back and said to him:

> "We're never going to talk about this again. I know you just got confused, and that little faggot got your head all twisted around. I don't want you to ever see him again. And as for what happened here today, it didn't happen. I don't want your mother to know

about this. No one will know about this, and you won't make this kind of mistake again. Do we understand each other?"

Rudy said he felt numb, as he nodded affirmatively, but never looking at his father. After that day, he became increasingly sad. He spent more and more time alone in his room. His mother noticed his dramatic downward spiral and attempted to ask him about it several times. Rudy just said it was nothing. She was convinced he was sick and took him to the family doctor for a physical. The doctor found no physical malady and suggested that Rudy was going through "the typical adolescent blues."

Four months later Rudy attempted to kill himself by slashing his wrists. His mother found him in the bathtub and called for immediate emergency assistance. After he was released from the hospital, Rudy was required to receive therapy to address the underlying psychological issues that had led up to his drastic course of action.

We met with Rudy alone and conducted several sessions with his family. For a long time Rudy didn't say much of anything. With time, he began to open up a little during our individual sessions together, but he remained guarded. It wasn't until 3 months had passed that Rudy finally explained to us why he wished he were dead. He told us about what had happened that fateful, tragic day with Jay and his father, and he told us he was a freak who didn't deserve to live.

Rudy had suffered terribly. As a gay male he had been subjected to horrible devaluation that came from both inside and outside of his family. Because of this devaluation, Rudy was deprived of a solid sense of community at all three levels. He felt like an alien in his family and at school. He had only one friend but felt he had to hide himself from even this person, which prevented the relationship from offering any genuine solace and support. Moreover, because of the stigma and violence directed against gays, Rudy was denied the opportunity to connect with other gay youth and have all the experiences that a normal adolescent is entitled to: dating; opportunities to talk with peers about love interests and troubles; the chance to see one's self reflected in movies, television shows, or magazines. A proliferation of homophobic and heterosexist forces had essentially prevented Rudy from experiencing a sense of cultural community in terms of his sexual orientation.

The alienation, fear, and shame Rudy had felt throughout most of his life were greatly intensified the day his father walked in on him and Jay. He lost many critical things on that day: his relationship with Jay; his relationship with his father (who barely looked at him after that); and even his relationship with his mother (while he had always felt close to her, the shame of this incident compelled him to distance himself from her). Rudy had also lost a piece of dignity and the hope that maybe he could finally acknowledge himself and stop hiding. All of these things were lost to him on that terrible day. Worst of all, none of these losses was recognized or acknowledged by anyone in his life. And where there is loss, there is rage. But for Rudy, his rage was buried deeply inside. The power of having his father so bluntly and brutally condemn him was deeply wounding. Rudy felt deep shame. And because Rudy had been so effectively socialized to believe there was something wrong with being gay, he believed that *he* was the problem. He believed he was sick and that he deserved the suffering he was feeling.

Our work with Rudy required us to help him begin to think about himself as normal and healthy, and to locate the problem where it truly resided—namely, outside of himself, in other people's bigoted, unjust hatred. The problem was not that Rudy was gay. Rather, the problem resided in others' attitudes about being gay. The problem was his father's homophobia. The problem was the homophobia and heterosexism of the surrounding world. We spent a lot of time softly challenging the idea that being gay is a problem. At one point we invited another gay teen into our sessions with Rudy. Martin was a very positive role model for Rudy. He was securely grounded in his identity and was able to speak with Rudy candidly and supportively about his experiences as a gay male, his struggles to come out, and how he had come to love himself. This was an important step because Martin's inclusion in the therapy process challenged the devaluation Rudy felt as a gay male, and it was a step toward helping him establish a positive sense of community with another gay male adolescent. It also was a critical step toward helping Rudy to realize that he had suffered terrible losses that were profoundly unjust. Martin disrupted the idea that gay was bad. Martin provided Rudy with a different way of thinking about himself. Once Rudy was able to entertain a different way of thinking about what his gayness meant, he could start to acknowledge that the losses he had suffered were unfair. It allowed him to relocate the source of his suffering. It was no longer that he was suffering because he was sick—he was suffering because other people's attitudes and beliefs were sick. With this cognitive shift, Rudy was gradually able to see his father's treatment of him as unfair and cruel. He was able to think about all the homophobic comments he had been exposed to over his lifetime as bigoted and cruel. He started to think about the alienation and shame he suffered from as symptoms of the meanness and injustice of the world around him rather than as symptoms of a sickness he carried within himself.

As Rudy began to think about the source of his pain differently, he was slowly able to recognize the cauldron of rage that he carried within himself. Gradually he became more and more aware of the rage he felt about the injustices to which he had been subjected. We helped Rudy to connect with his rage by asking him leading questions like "You've mentioned several times now that you're not convinced anymore that it's bad to be gay. If this is true, and it's not bad, then how do you make sense of what happened with your dad?"

Rudy answered that question by saying, "My dad doesn't understand about being gay. He was raised during a different time when people just assumed everyone was straight and had to be straight, so that's what he was raised to believe." This statement was critical because it marked a shift in Rudy's thinking about his identity. But also it's important to note Rudy's protectiveness of his father. He left his father a way out, and still didn't hold him accountable for his cruelty. At this point, Rudy still was not in touch with rage.

In cases where someone has difficulty gaining access to internalized rage, in addition to helping them shift cognitively so they think about their losses as unjust, we also actively work to give them permission to feel rage and to assure them that it is not necessarily a destructive force. Sometimes we directly say things like "What happened to you was unfair, and you're entitled to feel angry about this." Other times, as in Rudy's case, we are less direct and point out that it's possible to express anger toward someone and still love them. "You dad is your dad—of course, you love him. But it's possible to be mad at him for hurting you even though you love him."

Rudy responded to our statement with the first outward hint of rage we had ever seen from him. With his voice slightly raised he said, "Yeah, he has hurt me! He hasn't shown me much love, so maybe he doesn't deserve mine!"

This was a turning point in Rudy's healing process, because it was the first time he allowed himself to acknowledge even a hint of rage. Once we had that from him, we could move to the next step of encouraging him to "name his rage." We said to him, "How do you feel about the fact that your dad hasn't shown you much love?" Rudy finally said, "I'm mad at him." Once Rudy said that, his rage turned outward for the first time. It was now on the table where we could talk about it, examine it, and explore it directly.

Another phase of this work that was critical but we have under-stated here is what occurred with the family, especially Rudy's father. Working effectively with other parts of the family system is central to helping adolescents rechannel their rage. In the case of Rudy, the con-current work that we did with his family was necessary to facilitate his efforts to identify and express rage. It was just as important for his family to learn how to respond appropriately to his rage as it was for Rudy to be able to express it (appropriately). Also, having the entire family involved in the process enabled us to do the much-needed work devoted to the restoration of community.

"BEING WITH" AND VALIDATING RAGE

When adolescents begin to express their rage, those of us work-ing with them must find ways to "be with," and validate, their rage. In other words, we need to act as a container, as an emotional force field that is capable of holding and tolerating the intensity of their emotion. "Being with" rage is a form of nonreactive, active engagement. It requires emotional presence and attunement, but without emotional reactivity. When we are able to "be with" adolescents' rage, the mes-sage communicated indirectly is: "I'm here right by your side. I recog-nize what you're feeling, I understand, I'm feeling right along with you, and it's okay. I'm not threatened. I'm okay with what you're feel-ing. It's okay." This is the essence of "being with" an adolescents' rage. Similarly, it is necessary to validate the rage. A direct message must be communicated that says something akin to "You have a right to your rage—it makes sense that you feel this way." Unfortunately, there are few places where any of us, let alone adolescents, has per-mission to express rage. This is why demonstrating the ability to "be with and validate" rage is so vital. An essential part of helping adoles-cents learn to deal with their rage positively involves validating the legitimacy of rage.

For Rudy, admitting he was mad at his dad was his first overt, outward expression of rage, and with this first such admission the door was open. Subsequent to that he began to take more and more risks in therapy, verbalizing feelings of rage about the ways in which others' bigotry had affected his life. At first he expressed rage toward other youth, which was safe. Gradually, he began to express it toward his father, which was harder for him to do. At each step of the way, he witnessed the emergence of his voice and the rage that was a critical part of this voice. We validated this emotion repeatedly by telling him it was reasonable for him to feel this way. However, we also were cautious about the fact that, as a gay youth who had a virulently homophobic father, it was important to for him to be mindful of the responses he still might potentially receive from his dad. Our long-term goal, in cases like this one, is always to help the family and the adolescent find a way to coexist peacefully and respectfully. This is particularly poignant with gay and lesbian adolescents, because the risk of family rejection is extremely high. A disproportionate number of homeless teens in the streets of U.S. cities are gay teens who have been thrown out of their families simply because they are gay. Hence, in addition to validating Rudy's rage, we also relentlessly pointed out both the rewards and some of the inherent risks in his expressing it, particularly within his family. In fact, the silencing he endured in his family was one of the things he specifically expressed rage about in therapy.

CONNECTING LOSS, RAGE, AND VIOLENCE

Once rage is externalized and can be openly explored, it is critical to help adolescents make connections between loss, rage, and violence. The next task is to provide them with ongoing help in putting all of the pieces together so they can see how the different parts of their life experiences form a cohesive whole. A critical component of making the connections between loss, rage, and violence involves drawing out other more vulnerable emotions that are tied to loss and that underpin rage and violence. We have found that with some teens the best path to connecting loss, rage, and violence is by starting with loss and the vulnerable emotions associated with it, and building up to how these are related to rage and ultimately violence. With others, it tends to be easier to start with rage and then work back to loss and the vulnerable emotions underpinning rage and ultimately violence. Much of decision making regarding where to start is determined by where the adolescents are emotionally.

In Rudy's case the identification and acknowledgment of his losses set the stage for his beginning to connect consciously with rage. With the rehumanization of his loss, Rudy began to connect with the injustice that had been done to him, and this illuminated the rage that had been so deeply buried. Once this occurred, we were able to tie it all together with violence. For example, at one point we said to Rudy,

"You've had these very painful things that have happened to you, and now you're just starting to realize that you've had a lot of anger about this. But for all these years before you realized you had this anger, where did it go? Was it finding some way to get out without your knowing it?"

Initially, Rudy wasn't sure how he had been expressing his rage or his violence. Eventually, he started to piece together that he had found "hidden ways" of letting his rage out, meaning that he often made himself the target of his rage, which involved striking out against and hurting himself.

In Darryl's case, he had much more ready access to his rage and violence, but he struggled more to connect with his loss. In particular, he struggled with the vulnerable emotions that were hidden beneath his rage and ultimately his violence. To help him connect with these other emotions, we made statements such as: "It makes sense that you have anger about the many terrible things that have happened to you. But it also would make sense for you to have other types of feelings as well. What else do you think you feel besides anger?"

In Darryl's case, asking point-blank gave him the permission he seemed unable to give himself to acknowledge these other feelings. Certainly, not all adolescents open up so easily. When they don't, our recommendation is to hang in there, and persist gently and respectfully.

RECHANNELING RAGE

Ultimately, we want to assist adolescents in realizing that it's okay to feel rage in response to the pain and injustice of their losses. The critical issue involves what they do with their rage. *How and where* they channel their rage is what concerns us. We try to help them gain mastery over their rage so that they control it rather than their rage controlling them. We try to help them develop skills and strategies for harnessing and directing the power of their rage positively so that it shapes and creates rather than attacks and destroys. Finally, we believe that it is imperative that the rechanneling of rage should take place in socially sanctioned ways.

There is no singular formula for how to work with a given teen around the rechanneling of rage. Much of how this occurs depends upon the unique qualities and life circumstances of each adolescent, and of the person working with him or her. At best, we offer a general framework—a broad path that can be used as a guide in the adults' specific relationships with teens.

To effectively rechannel rage, it is necessary to have some idea about the unique interests and strengths of the adolescent in question. At the stage where it is reasonable to work on the rechanneling process, one should have ample information about the adolescent in question. It should be fairly easy to identify the types of things he or she is interested in and where his or her talents lie. This information provides the building blocks for the rechanneling process. Such information can be used to nurture and expand upon each adolescent's positive talents and interests as a way of rechanneling rage. Whether it's by encouraging a young person to pursue a passion for writing poetry, playing football, or becoming a photographer, it is vital to lend support that will enable adolescents to pursue their talents and interests. Artistic endeavors and athletics are especially common interest areas among adolescents, and they provide excellent vehicles for focusing and directing rage in constructive ways.

Sometimes the vehicle for rechanneling rage is something less obvious than an artistic or athletic interest. Consider Darryl, who never realized his own potential as a role model and advocate for the rights of abused and neglected children. As a young person who had felt the brutal pain of parental abandonment, and social indifference to his suffering, he identified deeply with children in similar circumstances. During several sessions with him we were consistently awed by the fire he displayed when referring to various children he had observed who had been mistreated by a parent and/or the community. He exhibited an intense awareness of young children and a deep empathy for their feelings. We realized this was a clue—this passion pointed toward a pathway that even Darryl was unaware of. We contacted a local community center that had a mentoring program in which older adolescents worked with and guided younger children. The adolescents, who were closely supervised by trained counselors, had difficult life experiences and a history of getting into trouble. The program was an opportunity for them to use their negative experiences in positive ways—to help transform themselves by using their troubles to guide younger children who might learn from them. Darryl was a natural for the program. It gave him a purpose—he felt needed. He was able to use his negative experiences for a positive purpose. He used his pain to help guide the children he mentored so they could learn from him.

Eventually, Darryl became more than a mentor. With the guidance and support of the center's director, Darryl eventually became involved in developing several programs for at-risk children. He became increasingly vocal as an advocate for children's rights. Working closely with the center's director, he spoke at several local events about his personal experiences and argued how important it was for parents, social service workers, and the community to invest more energy and resources in protecting children in need. Darryl had become an activist, and every time he argued on behalf of needy children he was using his rage constructively. He was drawing on the energy of his rage and using it to fuel his passionate advocacy on behalf of children at risk.

Rudy was another example of an adolescent who discovered an unexpected channel for his rage. Through his association with Martin, Rudy became introduced to an organization that supported the rights of gay youth. At first he joined the organization to receive much-needed support from a caring community. But, with time, Rudy started to get more involved in working with the organization to plan and carry out its various programs and initiatives. With time, Rudy became one of the organization's most committed and tireless workers. He wrote letters to and met with legislators, community leaders, school officials, and local business people about issues affecting gay youth. He eventually wrote a manual for gay youth that addressed the types of issues many confront in school and their families with respect to whether or not they should come out, how to handle reactions if and when they do, and where to turn to find support through all of this. In essence, Rudy was channeling his rage. He was using the fire inside, the fire that burned in response to pain and injustice, to achieve something positive. Rudy had learned to use his rage to work for him rather than against him.

Regardless of the type of channel an adolescent accesses, it should ultimately help him or her recognize that these activities are in fact a pathway for his or her rage. This connection must be made explicit. It is important to help adolescents become consciously aware of the relationship between their inner experience (e.g., feelings of pain and rage) and their outer experience or behaviors. We want them to see how everything is connected, because this is a vital aspect of disrupting the denial and disconnection that underpins many dysfunctional behaviors (e.g., substance abuse, aggression toward others). Second, we want them to consciously think about other positive actions as channels for their rage. Being mindful of their rage is a necessary dimension of having mastery over it. Moreover, we want adolescents to associate their feelings of rage with taking positive, concrete action. So, whenever they feel rage, we want them to form an instant association between their rage and some positive action. In Darryl's case, whenever he felt rage, he learned to instantly think about what he could do to work constructively as an advocate on behalf of at-risk children. Whenever Rudy felt his rage, he made an immediate association with how he could use his growing skills within his organization to support the rights of gay youth. In this way, both of them had achieved mastery of their rage and were using it as a force for positive change.

CHALLENGES OF WORKING WITH RAGE

Fear

Darryl, and those like him, is able to express rage much more freely than adolescents like Rudy. This can be a mixed bag for those working with violent and aggressive youth. On the one hand, ready access to rage makes the work we have to do a little less demanding. However, open expression of adolescent rage is not free of challenges. Fear poses the greatest obstacle to working effectively with rage. Inviting, being with, and validating rage are exceedingly difficult to do when feeling is overwhelmed by fear. Fear may be a response to a threat we perceive in relation to others' rage. As discussed in Chapter 5, we either fear the strong feelings that others' rage stirs within us and/or we fear that it will lead to violence—and, more specifically, violence against us. Consequently, to effectively help adolescents express their rage, we need to take basic steps to deal with our fear.

First, we need to assess whether an adolescent's rage is "out of control." In other words, does the person control the rage, or does it control the person? One way of making this assessment is by considering whether or not an adolescent's rage is being channeled physically. If an adolescent is physically lashing out (or threatening to lash out physically) against a person (self or others) or property, we tend to view this as an indicator that rage is out of control or threatening to get out of control. If there is no physical dimension associated with the expression of rage, we usually assess the risk of rage transforming into violence as fairly low.

The next step is to examine ourselves to determine how much of our fear is self-generated. In other words, does the fear stem more from an internal source than it does an externally based source? This is especially likely to be the case for anyone who has had negative experiences with others' rage. Anyone who has been injured, psychologically or physically, by another's rage is more prone to feeling threatened by it, even if the risk of violence is relatively low.

Those of us who have had traumatic experiences with rage, and are reactive to it, should strongly consider seeking support and, if necessary, therapy as a way of addressing levels of anxiety and discomfort that impede effective work with adolescents. It is nearly impossible to be helpful to violent and aggressive adolescents when there is a low tolerance level for expressions of rage. Therefore, targeted supervision or in some cases in-depth personal work regarding how to respond appropriately to rage may be necessary. Working intensively with violent youth and their strong emotions does require all of us to face our own inner demons before we can ever hope to be effective in assisting adolescents rechanneling rage.

The bottom line is that the presence of unmanaged fear compromises effectiveness. Granted no one of us can turn our fears on or off as we wish. However, it is important to have some awareness of the types of situations that invoke fear, as well as to know how we respond when this happens. Therefore, in situations where adolescents' rage ignites fear, we recommend finding ways to embrace it. Attempts to deny or ignore it are fruitless and counterproductive. Much as we believe rage must be confronted and addressed, we apply the same rule to fear. Therefore, when the response to adolescents' rage is fear, there are several steps we recommend taking as a way of coping with it. Since fear is almost always about feeling "out of control," what each of these steps share in common is that they are all ways of "taking control."

1. *Adjust the immediate external environment.* We believe that it only makes good common sense to thoroughly evaluate, for physical safety, the setting where most of the work with violent and aggressive adolescents will be conducted. The physical environment should be designed with angry, aggressive, and violent youth in mind. Practical decisions such as where offices and phones are located, which areas are secured and which are not, and even the specific physical arrangement of office furniture are all important factors to carefully consider. For example, in therapy situations we recommend prepositioning chairs in the room in a way that allows the therapist to sit nearest to the door. We also routinely work with teams behind the one-way mirror, which means the therapist is never truly alone with the client in different settings.

2. *Implement institutional remedies.* Those who work with adolescents in institutional settings should take steps to ensure that the issues of personal safety and emergency procedures have been addressed in a proactive, thoughtful, and comprehensive manner. For example, the locations where workers meet with adolescents should have access to phones that can be used to dial for emergency assistance. Doors to the premises should have locks that prevent outsiders from entering unannounced. Emergency procedures should be clearly posted and/or distributed to staff such that in the event of a crisis all staff members know who to call and other necessary measures to take to protect themselves appropriately. Ideally, on-site staff members who can provide support in a crisis situation should always be available.

3. *Address one's "inner environment."* We have hinted at this step throughout this chapter. We highlight it here to emphasize that there are both external and internal measures that can be employed to address fear. Addressing one's inner environment refers to the work that must occur within one's self. Anyone who works with adolescents must find ways to access their own level of comfort with intensity and with expressions of rage especially. For those who tend to consistently panic in the face of rage, professional intervention may be necessary as away of promoting one's own healing process. The goal is to be able to make adequate distinctions between rage that is reasonable versus rage that is in danger of crossing the line to violence. Learning skills for managing one's discomfort with rage is an important first step in having the presence of self and composure necessary to make such vital distinctions.

4. *Acknowledge one's fear directly.* This strategy involves disarming an adolescent's potentially violent rage by assuming a one-down position in response to it—for example, saying, "I have to be honest with you; I'm feeling a little uncomfortable now. The intensity of your rage is a little scary to me." We need to emphasize extreme caution with respect to assuming this position. In some cases it will work like a charm. Taking the "one-down" position soothes the adolescent's aggressive instinct, thereby pulling him or her "back from the edge." There are also situations, however, in which a show of vulnerability may have the opposite effect, that is, it may further arouse an adolescent's aggression and invite a full-scale attack. Unfortunately, there is no absolutely reliable method for discerning when this strategy is effective and when it should be avoided. It is extraordinarily helpful, however, to really know the adolescent before attempting it. Sometimes the best predictor of future behavior is past behavior. This strat-

egy, while an effective one, is not a maneuver that we recommend using during the early stages of a working relationship with violent and aggressive youth.

Parental Rage

Another common challenge of working with rage has to do with managing the rage that is sometimes experienced by parents or other family members. In families with teens who have had a lot of rage and/or who have acted violently, the entire system is under a great deal of stress. In some instances parents may become so fatigued and frustrated from trying to understand and cope with an enraged and/or aggressive adolescent that they become overwhelmed by their own underlying feelings of helplessness and exasperation. Having been unable to "break through" with their adolescent, some get to a point of resignation where they are ready to wash their hands of their teen and throw in the towel. In situations like these we commonly hear things like "We've done all we can do, we've had enough—he's your problem now" or "I'm at my wits end—I don't know what else to do, and frankly I'm tired of beating my head against a stone wall!"

Parents who may find themselves at the end of their proverbial rope often have a great deal of surface rage that masks deeper underlying feelings of helplessness and inadequacy. Many of them feel as though their adolescent's troubles are a reflection of their failure as parents. Rather than directly expressing their disappointment, many of them exhibit rage instead, like their children. This becomes problematic, because their rage makes it exceedingly difficult for them to interact with their adolescent in ways that are most beneficial. For example, in a therapy case consisting of a single-parent mother and a 14-year-old daughter, both exhibited high levels of rage. The daughter had been suspended from school for fighting, arrested for shoplifting, and routinely disobeyed her mother by sneaking out with friends and drinking. The daughter often snapped at her mother in therapy, and on one occasion she became so infuriated in a session that she threatened to throw a chair. The mother expressed that she was tired of her daughter's antics and said she didn't think she could take much more. She threatened to send her daughter to live with her sister and brother-in-law in California. The mother also expressed anger toward her daughter for her refusal to "shape up."

After several weeks of therapy the daughter started to respond, and minor improvements were evident in her behavior and demeanor.

However, when the therapist attempted to comment on these as way of encouraging the daughter, the mother became immediately reactive and enraged. She accused the therapist of being manipulated by the daughter. She insisted these changes were insincere and in reality the daughter was only "playing the therapist" so she could get out of therapy altogether. Unfortunately, the mother was so frazzled and angry about her extended struggles with her daughter, and the lack of progress she had become accustomed to, that she could not allow herself to have any faith in her daughter's recent efforts. Hence, the therapist not only had to work with the daughter's rage, he also had to work with the mother's rage, which was threatening to undermine the positive movement.

WORKING THROUGH RAGE WITH TIMOTHY, DAQUON, AND CARMEN

Timothy

Our work with Timothy required little from us in terms of *identifying and inviting expressions of rage*. He had almost instant access to his rage, and he expressed it in clearly discernible ways (e.g., yelling, using profanity, making hostile statements). However, Timothy seemed to have little sense of the roots of his rage. Early in our work together, we routinely asked him to talk about why he felt so angry. His responses were fairly superficial and lacked any acknowledgment of the deeper dynamics underpinning his strong emotions. While it is possible that Timothy had more self-awareness than he was letting on, our experience has suggested that most adolescents do not possess a comprehensive understanding of the anatomy of their rage. They are more likely to associate their rage with something that has just occurred at the moment, and are far less likely to see rage as the product of accumulated experiences with pain over a protracted period of time.

It was common for Timothy to "blow up" in therapy, lashing out at his parents, accusing them of being against him. Sometimes he lashed out at us, warning us to back off and leave him alone. During these occasions we worked assiduously to stay on course and validate his feelings. For instance, on one afternoon Timothy attended a session with his parents that started off in a volatile way. His parents having just found a stash of marijuana under his bed, both Timothy and his parents were furious with one another. Timothy resented that his mother had been "snooping in his room," and his parents were incensed to discover one more destructive thing he was doing.

The session began with Shaun lighting into Timothy, berating him for his delinquency and threatening to turn him over to the police. His mother interjected: "We're sick of this. Someone else is going to have to take over here, because we're fed up with you."

This was a pivotal moment. Our intervention, which consisted of *"being with" and validating the rage* in the room, was a key step in the work we had to do with rage. We started with a general statement: "Well, you're all very angry now, which makes sense, given what has happened." To his parents we said: "Clearly this latest incident has shattered some trust and some hope for you. Understandably you're feeling very threatened and helpless about what to do to help Timothy." To Timothy we said: "Of course, you must feel violated that your mom looked through your room. You're probably also feeling a lack of trust, and it makes sense this would make you very angry."

Early on in therapy we did a lot of this type of reflecting, "being with" and validating rage. Given the intensity of the emotion in this family, it was important to not move too quickly to dig deeper into what was under the rage. But eventually, as our trust grew, we did precisely that. We began probing into what was underneath the rage. This proved challenging at first, because in truth neither Timothy nor his parents really understood the roots of his rage. Timothy knew he felt relentless, all-consuming rage most of the time, and he knew he wanted to strike out at the world, but even he did not understand why. And in his quiet, self-reflective moments, when no one else could see him wrestling with himself, even he wondered why he had these destructive feelings. He even admitted to us once in session that he had brief moments where he scared himself. To assist Timothy in *connecting loss to rage and violence*, we said something similar to the following to him:

"You lost some important things when you were a little boy. Back before you grew into such a strong guy who is so good at defending himself, back when you were just a little guy who needed his dad, you got slammed with some pretty tough stuff. It had to be awful each and every time your dad abused you. And it had to be very upsetting when he left. Since you were just a little guy then, it probably all seemed like it was your fault, even though it wasn't. It had to be so confusing when one day, boom, he's gone and no one says anything to you. Then one day he's back and you're glad, but you start to wonder if he only came back because of Robert. And on top of that, he seemed so angry with you so much of the time, yelling at you and hitting you. All of this must have been sad and scary. I can see how you'd also feel really pissed off about that, and probably still do. It helps me understand now why you're so mad and why you've probably wanted to hurt your parents as much as they've hurt you. Heck, I can see why you would want to hurt anyone, just so long as you didn't have to keep feeling all those sad and bad feelings you have locked inside."

What we were doing with this statement was connecting loss with rage, and ultimately violence. Of course, stating the actual words did not render an immediate "Yes, that's it" from Timothy. But we did get an affirmative response nonetheless in the form of his silence. He neither said nor did anything; yet, we could feel that this was a different type of silence for him. It was a silence that was thick with the vulnerable emotions that underpin rage. We could sense that he was connecting with sadness, pain, and perhaps even shame.

Eventually we asked him what he was feeling. He shrugged his shoulders. We knew we were close to a breakthrough, but we also knew that if we weren't careful, we would scare him and he would retreat back into his fortress and slam the door in our face.

"It could just be our craziness, Timothy, but if we had to guess, we'd say you were feeling sad right now. And if you are, we want you to know it's okay. In fact, we think it takes a lot of courage to feel sad. Most guys aren't strong enough to be able to admit when they feel sad."

He continued to sit there in silence.

"So, can you tell us what it was like for you when you were a little boy and your dad yelled at you for the smallest things, and punched and hit you? What was it like when he left? How did you feel? And what was it like when he came back and you thought it was because of Robert and not you?

"It sucked," he finally retorted. "It made me want to hurt him as much has he was hurting me."

There it was! In his own words, Timothy was acknowledging his pain and making the connection between his pain, rage, and violence. What we were able to do then, after validating what he had expressed, was to amplify this connection by stating, "So, that's when you first learned that when you feel hurt or sad, to cover it up by getting angry and lashing out." From that point forward, any time Timothy expressed rage and intimated violence, we translated this into "You're feeling hurt and sad now—that's the reason for all the rage and violence."

Now that we had expanded the meaning of rage such that it was a sign that Timothy was feeling hurt and sad, we had a way of normalizing his emotion. Now his rage wasn't just an irrational, out-of-control explosion that made him look "crazy" to others. Rather, it was evidence of some injustice and pain that he had suffered. With that established, we could explain to Timothy that his rage made sense—it was reasonable given what he had experienced—but also, how he handled his rage was important. We explained the difference between having mastery over one's rage versus it mastering you. This frame was especially effective with a teen like Timothy who was highly invested in "being in control." Since he wanted to appear cool and in control, we had set up a situation in which the only way he could do that was by exercising some authority over his rage. To do this, we needed to develop *constructive ways of rechanneling rage.*

One of the things that Timothy expressed a strong interest in was football. He had a desire to play from the time he was quite young, but his mother was afraid of his getting injured. At best, this was a tricky issue. We encouraged his parents to weigh the potential risks of his playing (and perhaps sustaining an injury but potentially finding a constructive way to channel his energies and positively relate to peers) with his not playing (and not developing a constructive way of channeling his energy, in which case he was likely to continue with his destructive methods of channeling). Kate remained skeptical, although Shaun was strongly in favor of the idea.

After a great deal of discussion, the Ryans finally consented to allow Timothy to try out for his high school football team. Much to Timothy's delight he made the varsity team. During his first season his playing time was not as much as he would have liked it to be. Despite numerous early threats to quit, he stayed on the team, and there was a noticeable difference in his moods. By the end of his first season, he seemed a little more focused and less volatile. His place on the football team fostered the creation of an extended community for Timothy, and it also provided him with a vehicle for channeling some of the rage he had been carrying. Moreover, the affirming feedback he started to receive from peers about his athletic skills played a critical role in challenging the devaluation that plagued him.

Daquon

Identifying and inviting rage proved to be a far greater challenge with Daquon than with Timothy. Daquon's entire demeanor was crafted to hide any overt, obvious expression of rage. It was all part of his "cool posing." Since he wasn't about to openly *identify and acknowledge his rage*, we had to engage in *tracking, validating, and zooming.* For example, we closely tracked Daquon's story of how he had been sent back to the youth center for a crime he hadn't committed. We responded with validation by saying that we thought this was terribly unfair. He nodded in agreement. With that we began to zoom in by saying, "What effect has it had on you to be the victim of such an injustice?"

Because Daquon did not reveal rage easily, he responded guardedly: "It made me hard and it made me smart. I don't have any false beliefs about justice. I accept reality, and I've had to get myself ready to deal with this stuff. I'm a survivor."

While Daquon guarded against revealing his rage, we persisted, continuing to track, validate, and zoom in. "You are a survivor. The blows you've been hit with and the fact that you're still here are a testimonial to your skills as a survivor. And we're also appreciating the fact that it has to take a lot of energy to survive, and it doesn't leave much time for anything else . . . like just enjoying life."

"That's a luxury no black man in America has. We weren't put here to enjoy life . . . that's for white boys," he retorted.

"You're right, black men definitely do not have the privileges that white men have . . . including the freedom to walk outside your front door and not have to constantly watch your back. So, what do you think about this? Do you think this is fair?"

"Hell, no, it's not fair."

"And how do you feel when you see something that is unfair or unjust?"

"I don't like it."

"But how does it make you feel?"

"Mad."

At last, there was some small movement. We understand that indicating that he was mad was only one small step toward recognizing rage. Now we could begin to move in gradually and encourage him to take the emotional journey from mad to rage. We continued to help him move closer to his rage, knowing at some point he would actually express it with greater intensity and frequency. Once he did, we understood that we would need to nonreactively *"be with" and validate the rage.*

Next we turned to *connecting loss, rage, and violence.* In Daquon's case, he knew that he was filled with rage, and he had some understanding of why. He also had some sense of how all of this was connected to his propensity for violence. But what he lacked was the opportunity to express any of this in an uncensored, uncalculated way. Moreover, he was disconnected from the vulnerable emotions that resided beneath his rage. To get at all of this, we devoted our efforts to addressing Daquon's losses. We started in the place where he was comfortable, engaging with his loss cognitively. He was able to name most of his losses to us and describe them in an emotionally frozen way. Initially we went along with this. But eventually we started to push deeper. With the aid of the loss diagram we were able to graphically depict his loss story, which had a visibly unsettling effect on him. When we asked him about this, he explained, "I guess I knew a lot of things have happened to me, but when you put that thing together like that, it's even more than I thought. It's a lot."

When Daquon uttered the words "It's a lot," we were on the verge of moving from a cognitive acknowledgment of loss to an emotional one.

"Yes, it *is* a lot, especially for someone so young. How does it make you feel when you see this and realize how much you've lost in your short life?"

"It makes me mad."

He quickly moved to rage to avoid the more vulnerable emotions that were starting to bubble up.

"Okay, it makes you mad. What else? There's more."

"Just mad, okay."

His rage was beginning to brew . . . a defensive response against the pain he was starting to feel. But we kept pushing.

"Yeah, you keep saying mad, but your face is saying something else."

"Jesus Christ! What the hell do you want from me?" He was screaming now.

"We just want to know what's under all that rage. Can you tell us, 'cause we can see you're feeling something else."

"Just go to hell! . . . Leave me alone!"

But, as these words came spitting out, a single tear also escaped and rolled down his cheek. It seemed to stun him, and for a moment it looked as if he might try to pretend it hadn't happened, but then he seemed to realize it was too late. It was out—there was no point in holding it back anymore. He choked on the deep sobs that began to reverberate through his body while he buried his face in his hands as if to hide the tears that were spilling out. He seemed ashamed.

With this breakthrough we were able, at last, to talk with Daquon openly about his loss and pain as well as his rage. He listened a lot, and we continued to make vital connections. It was important to help him understand the depth of his loss and how few opportunities he had had to experience his pain and grief. It also was important to help him understand how he'd been conditioned to deny feelings of pain, which only intensified his rage, which was a precursor to his violence.

Because Daquon had a strong connection with his identity as a black male, we were able to capitalize on this by pointing out how his denial of his emotions, especially of his pain, only reinforced his oppression as a black male. Since the very beginning of slavery in the Americas, white racism has sought to repress all emotion in black people as a way of intensifying their objectification. Hence, one way for Daquon to resist racism was by embracing his humanness through acknowledging and experiencing his own emotions. It was a frame to which he could relate. Yet, we also were realistic about the fact that while it was in his best interests to be connected to his feelings, he needed to exercise good judgment about when and how he expressed himself. Specifically, we worked on helping him to develop *strategies for rechanneling his rage positively*: we encouraged him to use rage as a tool for transformation rather than a weapon of destruction.

Daquon's passion for racial justice turned out to play a vital role in the rechanneling of his rage. In therapy we actively encouraged his sense of racial consciousness and often praised his keen racial critiques and his intense commitment to black liberation. It was his *gift for giving*. We also pointed out how the world and his community needed someone like him—that there was a lot of work for him to do and he could ill afford to make unintelligent choices that would only undermine his opportunity to use his talents for a greater good. We explained how important it was for him to think beyond himself and to keep his "eyes on the prize." As we had these conversations with him, what we discovered was that he had a secret fantasy about becoming a civil rights attorney, but he never believed this was a real possibility for himself. We strongly nurtured this aspiration and assisted him in developing a realistic plan for how he could get into college and begin his journey toward his goal.

We were realistic with him and acknowledged that he was going to face further injustices along the way that would be designed to discourage him, but his task was to keep his "eyes on the prize" and never give up—to not be deterred, to remember what was at stake. In the interim, we facilitated a connection between him and a successful African American attorney who agreed to take Daquon under his wing and mentor him. At first Daquon was reticent, saying this would be too much of a hassle, but he took the challenge on and eventually came to love it. He was well on his way to finding a vehicle for rechanneling his rage in a positive manner that would allow him to be a force for justice and healing. Of course, as is always the case with adolescents like Daquon, Timothy, and the countless others we have yet to meet, it is a day-to-day process.

Carmen

The process of *identifying and inviting rage* from Carmen was extremely challenging. On the surface, she exhibited no obvious sign of rage. Her overall demeanor was one of depression. Yet, we knew that, deep down inside, Carmen carried a great deal of rage, and our first task was to unearth it and bring it forth. While to the casual observer it would have seemed bizarre to even speak of rage, we have found that with teens like Carmen one of the best ways to uncover rage that has been turned inwardly is to come right out and name it. For example, with Carmen we said the following:

"I know you say you are depressed, and you certainly look depressed, but we have this crazy idea about you—that there's more going on inside than meets the eye. We think that what you're feeling, in addition to sadness, is anger. In fact, we think you're feeling rage, but, for whatever reason, you aren't comfortable showing this feeling. So, instead, you've turned in all inside. It's like your feelings are folding in on you, like your rage is being sucked down inside you into quicksand and it's gotten buried deep in your gut where it's hard to see on the outside, but it's there."

Carmen listened to our disclosure politely, and then she denied having any such emotion. Yet, we saw a flicker in her eye. It was a faint connection—something was registering inside. However, she wasn't ready yet to acknowledge rage. After all, she had buried it for a reason—because it was too scary for her to admit, even to herself. Our one push in this direction wasn't going to change that in one session, but it was a start. For the next several sessions, whenever Carmen spoke we continued to introduce the theme of rage. We continued to suggest that it would make sense for her to feel rage in light of what she was sharing, and we remained curious about where rage might be hiding if it wasn't out in the open.

Because her rage was so deeply buried, we had to use our *tracking, validating, and zooming-in* skills. We listened closely for any hint of rage, and when he heard it we validated and zoomed in on it. For example, several weeks after we first introduced rage, Carmen came to a session looking more animated than we'd ever seen her. She started by saying she had just come from her hairstylist, where she'd had an appointment for a trim. During her appointment the stylist had suggested that Carmen try something really different—like coloring her hair blond. "I can't believe she would suggest that to me!" Carmen said with indignation.

We followed her indignation, knowing where it was likely to lead. "Why can't you believe it?" we asked.

"Because it's insulting. Like she thinks that somehow I'm not good enough with my dark hair . . . like everyone naturally wants to be blonde because somehow that's better. I'm sick of this." We validated her sense of indignation and zoomed in by asking her to tell us more about what she thought the stylist's comments were reflective of and why that was so insulting to her. "I guess I'm just tired of people in this country acting as if blond hair, blue eyes, and white skin is the only thing that is good or beautiful. How do you think that makes someone like me feel?"

"Well, we have an idea . . . but can you tell us for yourself how it makes you feel?"

"It makes me angry. I'm tired of this—tired of never feeling good enough. I've been thinking a lot about what you said to me about my being enraged, and more and more I am thinking that maybe you are right."

Finally Carmen was acknowledging her own rage. Our job then was to invite more of it and to really encourage her to let it out. And as she did, we were right there by her side, *"being with" and validating her rage.* We also encouraged her to explore and discuss her thoughts about how she had learned to bury her anger and rage—what messages had she received along the way that made these feelings so taboo? We were gradually helping her to make vital connections between loss and rage by uncovering the ways in which she felt rage in response to her losses, and how one of the things she had lost was her freedom to even acknowledge, express, and embrace her rage. The silencing that had occurred with respect to her rage was yet another loss—and it had been a costly loss at that. With the silencing of her rage, the energy of it had finally imploded inside of Carmen, and the effect had been the string of self-destructive behaviors she had inflicted upon herself—she became the reliable target of her own rage turned to violence. For Carmen, finally seeing the relationship between her loss, rage, and violence was a turning point. It had a transformative effect on her emotional disposition. All that had been turned inwardly and that was dragging her down was released, and with this release the young woman who had been incarcerated was leaving her cell. We started to see a newly emerging sense of power in Carmen.

With the expression of her rage and the understanding of how it typically led to violence against herself, she began to discover a restless passion deep within. This newly found spirit of fire made her want to speak about injustices she had suffered and to become a voice in support of the liberation of women of color. As a talented writer, Carmen started *rechanneling her rage* by writing for the school newspaper. She wrote several powerful articles about the political crisis in South American countries and the role the United States had played in undermining true independence and democracy in those nations. She also wrote about the effects of racism and sexism on the identity development of girls of color, using her own story as a primary vehicle. These articles led her to a network of other women of color at her school who offered social support and much-needed community, as well as opportunities to further rechannel rage through meaningful social and political activism.

CONCLUSION

Rage is a normal, healthy response to pain and injustice. Those who suffer from devaluation, the disruption or community, and the dehumanization of loss will inevitably experience rage. When rage is suppressed and/or denied, eventually it will explode and lead to violence, either inwardly or externally. To prevent this from occurring, effective rage work is necessary, which involves identifying and inviting rage; "being with" and validating it; understanding connections between loss, rage, and violence; and developing constructive ways of rechanneling rage.

CHAPTER 11

• • • • • • • •

Final Reflections

We live in a world of violence. For some of us the violence lives in our homes. At times we are the targets, assaulted by the fists of abusive partners. At times we are the violent ones, lashing out at our children or our elderly parents. For some of us the violence flourishes just outside of our front doors. Sometimes it follows us while we walk down the street, and sometimes it speeds around the corner in a spray of bullets fired from the gun of a drive-by shooter. The violence can be found in our schools, in our places of work, in the malls where we shop, the airports and train stations we pass through, and the neighborhoods where we live. It enters the spaces of our lives when we send off loved ones to fight on the frontlines of a war zone on the other side of the globe. It permeates our lives through the television and computer screens that project images of destruction carried out by terrorists whose violence is enabled by their resolve about death, and by everyday people whose violence is fueled by their fear of death.

We live in a world of violence—whether it's the violence committed by loved ones, by faceless strangers, or by the brutality of poverty, racism, sexism, and homophobia. There is no escape from the violence. And this may be the greatest challenge we face in our work to prevent adolescent violence and to help our young people heal from the violence they have endured. We are faced with the seemingly impossible task of trying to teach our young people that violence is not an answer, while so much of what they see in the world suggests otherwise. There is a complicated tension that exists between what we tell adolescents to do and what the realities of our world convey to them. How do we promote peace when there is so much violence?

In this book we have presented a way of thinking about and addressing adolescent violence that is rooted in a systemic orientation. By counteracting devaluation, restoring community, rehumanizing loss, and rechanneling rage, we believe it is possible to make steady progress in promoting nonviolence in the lives of our young people. But it is essential to recognize and address the interrelatedness of all four aggravating factors. It is not enough to focus attention on one or two of the factors. Rather, it is vital to see how all four coexist, to attend to the synergistic interplay among them. This is what it means to adopt a systemic orientation, which is critical in achieving positive change.

As we have endeavored to underscore, a central part of utilizing a systemic orientation involves seeing the connection between any number of things that may appear unrelated but nonetheless are very much related. Throughout this book we have argued that it is necessary to see the connection that exists between what happens at the micro level (the little picture) and the macro level (the big picture). This means seeing and addressing the tension that is created when we advocate nonviolence on a direct, personal level but remain oblivious to manifestations of violence on the broader scale, as if somehow poverty, racism, homophobia, sexism, and war are not expressions of violence that have devastating effects.

The systemic orientation we have presented in this book calls for an integrated approach to understanding and addressing violence. While we stand by the many strategies we have presented, in and of themselves they are essentially useless. Our approach to addressing adolescent violence is less about a grab bag of strategies and more about a way of seeing the world, a way of being. As such, our efforts must begin with recognizing our relatedness to all life on our planet. At the risk of sounding melodramatic, we do believe that the earth is a system and what happens in one part affects what happens in all the rest. As such, we simply cannot afford to tolerate suffering in some other family, neighborhood, or nation under the false premise that "that's their problem, not mine." We are all connected, so what happens to "other(s)" eventually comes back to oneself. With this as our underlying orientation, we hope above all else that we have inspired readers to see the connections that exist among all things, which begins with looking closely at ourselves and recognizing the tension that sometimes exists between our beliefs and our behaviors.

We believe it is imperative to recognize and strive to resolve the tension that often exists between the values we preach and the actual actions we take. Specifically, it is necessary to recognize the tension that is generated when we say violence is wrong but engage in or support violent behaviors. In fact, many of us do not even recognize this tension because we have learned how to rationalize our behaviors so that it appears as if our actions "are not really violence" or are somehow "acceptable violence." Whether it's the parent who says "I hit him for his own good—to teach him," or the person who argues that "war is necessary because we have to get them before they get us," or the person who defends eating the flesh of animals because "that's why they're here—for us to eat," these are all classic rationales that we teach our children. The message we are sending is that violence is wrong *unless* it's for the purpose of teaching a lesson that is for the recipients' own good, or unless it's a matter of doing unto others *before* they do unto you, or unless the target of the violence is somehow less than you—less intelligent, less moral, less spiritual, less of anything that you consider a criterion for being treated with dignity and respect.

The examples of how we use common rationalizations to justify our own violence are countless. Rationales like these were used to by white Europeans to justify the genocide of Native Americans and the enslavement of Africans. For centuries men employed similar rationales to justify the subjugation of women, including denial of the right to own property, to vote, and to make decisions about their own bodies. Many of us employ these rationales to justify economic oppression, violence against gays, lesbians, and bisexuals, religious persecution, and the brutal treatment of animals who are exploited for food, entertainment, and experimentation. And all too often many of us use these rationales to justify responding to the violence of adolescents with punishment and domination, which is all about violence. These rationales reside at the heart of the tension that often exists between our broader commitment to nonviolence and the specific ways that our actions support violence. At the start of this book we suggested that rationales like these, while convenient, are dangerous, because they send a mixed message to young people. It teaches them how to become proficient in rationalizing, not relinquishing, their violence.

Adolescents are excellent observers of the adult world and they hear our rhetoric about nonviolence, but they also see the reality of our actions and they learn to employ the same rationales we employ to justify their actions. Throughout this book we offered many examples of young people who skillfully rationalized their own violence. Herein lies the need for a systemic orientation. If we are truly to reach young people and to positively transform their lives, we need to closely scrutinize ourselves as our point of departure.

Looking within at ourselves is hard. It's never easy to self-reflect and to place one's own behaviors under the microscope. In our own lives both of us have struggled immensely with this challenge. As this book attests, we have a lot to say about challenging violence and promoting kinder, gentler ways of relating. Yet, we too have our own tensions between what we believe and how we behave. Through intentional effort we have made progress to ease these tensions, but even now the work remains unfinished. This is a point we cannot stress enough! the work to "stop the violence" is hard work and it is constant work. Because we live in a world of violence, purity—at least for most of us—is impossible. Tension between what we preach and what we practice will remain present to some degree for most of us. Nonetheless we believe each of us must work vigilantly to ease this tension, to always strive to do better than we are doing, and to remain honest with ourselves and others about the reality of how well we are doing.

Finally, in this book we have tried to offer a way of thinking about adolescents who are violent as hurt rather than as bad. This perspective is paramount in our work with violent adolescents. If we are to prevent and heal the violence in the lives of our young people, it starts with shifting how we see them. While it is all too easy to see the ugliness of their behaviors, it is much harder to see the hurt that lies beneath. But seeing the hurt is a necessary part of feeling the compassion that is an antidote for our own impulse to want to lash out, to dominate, to punish, and to resort to aggression. Just as we want them to resist the urge to violence, we too must resist this urge, and it starts with shifting how we think about and understand adolescents who are violent.

The various components of our model all work together to humanize adolescents who are violent so that we can see the suffering beneath their violence. Seeing adolescents as hurt rather than bad is essential to successfully addressing and ultimately preventing adolescent violence. This is in essence what we have tried to present in this book. And as we have said many times, ultimately all of this depends on who we are and on our ability to be self-reflective, honest, and willing to challenge ourselves to live our own lives in greater harmony with the values of peace and nonviolence. Through our own efforts to live more congruently, and to strive constantly to do better, ourselves, we increase our capacity to see adolescents who are violent in humanized ways, which helps us to respond to them with the compassion and wisdom that they deserve.

References

Alderman, T. (1997). *The scarred soul: Understanding and ending self-inflicted violence*. Oakland, CA: New Harbinger.

Allen, E. (1994, July). Missing children: A fearful epidemic. *USA Today Magazine*.

Bell, C. (1991). Traumatic stress in children in danger. *Journal of Health Care for the Poor and Undeserved, 2*, 175–188.

Centers for Disease Control and Prevention. (1997). Rates of homicide, suicide, and firearm related death among children—26 industrialized countries. Morbidity and Mortality Weekly Report, *46*(5).

Centers for Disease Control and Prevention. (1998). *Youth Risk Behavior 16 Surveillance—United States, 1997*. Washington, DC: U.S. Department of Health and Human Services.

Cooley-Quille, M. R., Turner, S. M., & Beidel, D. C. (1995). Emotional impact of children's exposure to community violence: A preliminary study. *Journal of the American Academy of Child and Adolescent Psychiatry*, 1362–1368.

Garbarino, J. (1995). *Raising children in a socially toxic environment*. San Francisco: Jossey-Bass.

Garbarino, J. (1999). *Lost boys: Why our sons turn violent and how we can save them*. New York: Free Press.

Garbarino, J. & Delara, E. (2003). *And words can hurt forever: How to protect adolescents from bullying, harassment, and emotional violence*. New York: Simon & Schuster.

Garrett, A. G. (2003). *Bullying in schools: Causes, preventions, and interventions*. McFarland & Company.

Gordon, R. A. (1990). *Anorexia and bulimia: Anatomy of a social epidemic*. New York: Blackwell.

271

Hampton, R. L., Jenkins, P., & Gullotta, T. P. (1996). *Preventing violence in America*. Thousand Oaks, CA: Sage.

Hardy, K. V. (1997, January). Not quite home: The psychological effects of oppression. *In the Family*, pp. 7–9; 25–27.

Hardy, K. V. (1999). *Bullies to buddies program*. New York: Ackerman Institute for the Family.

Imber Black, E. & Roberts, J. (1993). *Rituals for our times: Celebrating, healing, and changing our lives and our relationships*. New York: Harpercollins.

Karr-Morse, R., & Wiley, M. S. (1997). *Ghosts from the nursery: Tracing the roots of violence*. New York. Atlantic Monthly Press.

Kozol, J. (1991). *Savage inequalities*. New York: HarperCollins.

Kübler-Ross, E. (1970). *On death and dying: What the dying have to teach doctors, nursers, clergy, and their own families*. New York: Macmillian.

Laszloffy, T. A. (2000). Awesome allies. *Family Therapy Networker*, Jan./Feb., 71–81.

Lewis, D. O. (1992). From abuse to violence: Psychophysiological consequences of maltreatment. *Journal of American Academy of Child and Adolescent Psychiatry, 31*(3), 383–391.

Majors, R., & Mancini-Billson, J. (1992). *Cool pose: The dilemmas of black manhood in America*. New York: Simon & Schuster.

Nunnally, E. & Moy, C. (1989). *Communication basics for human service professionals, Vol. 56*. Thousand Oaks: CA: Sage Publications.

Office of Juvenile Justice and Delinquency Prevention. (1997). *Juvenile offenders and victims: 1997 update on violence*. Washington, DC: U.S. Department of Justice.

Olweus, D. (1993). *Bullying at school: What we know and what we can do (Understanding children's worlds)*. Blackwell Publishing.

Pipher, M. (1994). *Reviving Ophelia*. New York: Grossett/Putman.

Pollack, W. (1998). *Real boys: Rescuing our sons from the myths of boyhood*. New York. Holt.

Rubin, L. (1992). *Worlds of pain*. New York: Basic Books.

Satir, V. (1972). *Peoplemaking*. Palo Alto, CA: Science and Behavior Books, Inc.

Selekman, M. & O'Hanlon, B. (2002). *Living on the razor's edge*. W. W. Norton.

Shervington, W. W. (2000). We can no longer ignore the rising rate of African American suicide. *Journal of the American Medical Association, 92*(2), 53–54.

Shisslak, C. M., Crago, M., & Estes, L. S. (1995). The spectrum of eating disturbances. *International Journal of Eating Disorders, 18*(3), 209–219.

Snyder, H. N. (2000). *Special analyses of FBI serious violent crimes data*. Pittsburgh: National Center for Juvenile Justice.

Snyder, H., & Sickmund, M. (1999). *Juvenile offenders and victims: 1999 national report*. Washington, DC: Office of Juvenile Justice and Delinquency Prevention.

Taffel, R., & Blau, M. (2001). *The second family: How adolescent power is challenging the American family*. New York: St. Martin's Press.

Thornberry, T., & Burch, J. (1997). *Gang members and delinquent behavior.* Washington, DC: Office of Juvenile Justice and Delinquency Prevention.

U.S. Department of Health and Human Services, Administration on Children, Youth and Families (2003). *Child welfare outcomes 2000: Annual report.* Washington, DC: U.S. Government Printing Office.

Walker, A. (1989). *The temple of my familiar.* New York: Washington Square Press.

Walsh, F. (1998). *Strengthening family resilience.* New York: Guilford Press.

Wessler, S. & Preble, W. (2003). *Respectful schools: How educators and students can conquer hate and harassment.* Washington, DC: Association for Supervision and Curriculum Development.

Wisdom, C. S. (1992, October). *The cycle of violence: National Institute of Justice research in brief* (MJ 136607), Washington, DC: U.S. Department of Justice. pp. 1–6.

Wolf, N. (1997). *Promiscuities: The secret struggle for womanhood.* New York: Ballantine.

Index